MRI/CT AND PATHOLOGY IN HEAD AND NECK TUMORS
A Correlative Study

SERIES IN RADIOLOGY

VOLUME 18

MRI/CT and Pathology in Head and Neck Tumors

A Correlative Study

With 230 Photographs

ROLAND CHISIN

MARK W. RAGOZZINO / MICHAEL P. JOSEPH / ALFRED L. WEBER
MAX L. GOODMAN / RICHARD L. FABIAN

Edited by
ROLAND CHISIN

Foreword by
JACQUELINE VIGNAUD

Editorial Advisor
ALFRED L. WEBER

Kluwer Academic Publishers
DORDRECHT – BOSTON – LONDON

Library of Congress Cataloging in Publication Data

MRI/CT and pathology in head and neck tumors.
     (Series in radiology, volume 18)
     1. Head—Tumors—Diagnosis. 2. Neck—Tumors—Diag-
nosis. 3. Head—Magnetic resonance imaging. 4. Neck—Magnetic
resonance imaging. 5. Head—Tomography. 6. Neck—Tomography. I. Chisin, Roland, 1947–   . II. Weber, Alfred L. III.
Series. [DNLM: 1. Head and Neck Neoplasms—pathology. 2.
Head and Neck Neoplasms—radiography. 3. Magnetic Resonance Imaging. 4. Tomography, X-Ray Computed.
WE 707 M939]   RC280.H4M75   1989   616.99′2910757
89–2474

ISBN-13: 978-94-010-6916-8   e-ISBN-13: 978-94-009-0947-2
DOI: 10.1007/978-94-009-0947-2

Published by Kluwer Academic Publishers,
P.O. Box 17, 3300 AA Dordrecht, The Netherlands.

Kluwer Aademic Publishers incorporates
the publishing programmes of
D. Reidel, Martinus Nijhoff, Dr W. Junk and MTP Press.

Sold and distributed in the U.S.A. and Canada
by Kluwer Academic Publishers,
101 Philip Drive, Norwell, MA 02061, U.S.A.

In all other countries, sold and distributed
by Kluwer Academic Publishers Group,
P.O. Box 322, 3300 AH Dordrecht, The Netherlands.

To my late father,
to my wife Sylvie, and
to my children Yoram and Caroline,
in appreciation for their encouragement,
patience and sacrifice.

ROLAND CHISIN

Foreword

Over the past 60 years, radiology has progressively uncovered the human body. At first a fleshless skeleton for global study, the body then appeared in slices, until with present techniques its smallest structures are revealed. The physician at the computer console is constantly amazed at the never-ending series of organ sections and their multiple images arising through manipulation of the signal. Cerebral convolutions, orbital content, bone marrow, the face and all its bones can now be made visible without any danger to the patient. A lesion can be detected, located and identified; it can be observed in sections of multiple orientation, and reconstructed in three dimensions; contours can be given, and coordinates calculated in relation to a reference point allowing manual or automatic stereotactic intervention.

CT (Computerized Tomography) and MRI (Magnetic Resonance Imaging) are among the most important techniques for imaging the human body. Between them, these two techniques generate large amounts of quantitative and qualitative data. In order to acquire informative value, these data must be processed by the human brain. For this a frame of reference is indispensable.

In any imaging procedure, the morphology of the structures shown is recognized by comparing them with anatomy, whether normal or pathological. CT and MRI are excellent for this purpose: comparison of the images with anatomic sections allows identification of all macroscopic structures. Tissue characterization is approached via microscopic anatomy and analysis of phenomena which result from the interaction between magnetic fields and matter. Even today, this interaction is often not fully understood, and the ways to demonstrate it by different MRI pulse sequences are not always evident.

The results of these imaging procedures cannot be interpreted in isolation. For the progress of diagnos-

tic knowledge, a multidisciplinary approach is indispensable: clinicians, radiologists, surgeons, radiotherapists, and pathologists must all contribute their respective inputs for every patient referred. Moreover, experience is acquired through knowledge of cases whose diagnosis is certain, and with which new cases can be compared. In this way a data base is created, whether in the physician's memory or in that of the computer, which is helpful in making diagnoses.

Dr. Roland Chisin, who is both an otolaryngologist and a biophysicist, is well qualified to write and edit a volume such as this, and this book will undoubtedly find its place in the overall effort, perhaps as the first pages of a thesaurus for use in the diagnosis of head and neck tumors.

The 35 cases selected are representative for tumor pathology in the field of otorhinolaryngology. They are all well documented, clinically, radiologically and pathologically. The comments are precise: they address the techniques and compare the contributions of MR and CT images to morphology and tissue characterization whenever the latter is possible. The study of these 35 cases, the iconography of which is excellent, will be of great use to the student and also to the experienced radiologist and otolaryngologist wishing to learn the radiological signs of these tumors. Moreover, the different parameters can be used as the embryo of a database bank, as suggested in the concluding remarks.

In the chapter before the concluding remarks, which is in fact the book's summing-up, the place of MRI among the imaging techniques for the different regions of the extracranial head and neck is discussed. These reflections are also relevant to the cost/efficiency problem of determining the algorithm which will yield the most precise diagnosis.

The studies and discussions on which this book is

based were carried out in Boston through the collaborative efforts of teams from Harvard Medical School, Massachusetts Eye and Ear Infirmary, and Massachusetts General Hospital.

It was in Boston that Dr. Harold Schuknecht carried out his authoritative work. This book is written in the same spirit and with the same rigor.

Paris, 8 September 1989   Dr. Jacqueline Vignaud

Contents

Contents

Acknowledgements

The authors wish to acknowledge with gratitude the contributions of the following persons:

Mrs. Karen M. Lane, who is the Research Administrator of the Department of Radiology at the Massachusetts Eye and Ear Infirmary, Boston, Massachusetts. Without her unflagging dedication, exceptional organizational talent, and editorial and typing skills, this book would not have been possible.

Yael Segal and Dorothy Vaddai of the Department of Medical Biophysics and Nuclear Medicine, Hadassah Hospital, Jerusalem, for their help in the typing and editing of the manuscript, and Esther Cameron for editorial final touches.

Paul Beaulieu, Mary Ann Kotowski, Nancy Yourkewicz and Ellen Block, NMR Technologists at the MRI Section of the Massachusetts General Hospital, Boston, Massachusetts, who carried out most of the tests on which this book is based.

The dedicated team of the Photolaboratory at the Massachusetts Eye and Ear Infirmary and Stephen Conley of the Pathology Photolaboratory at the Massachusetts General Hospital, who provided the photographs.

Dr. Thomas J. Brady, Head of MRI at the Massachusetts General Hospital, for his tremendous help and encouragement.

Dr. Bruce Rosen, Clinical Director of MRI at the Massachusetts General Hospital, for his judicious comments concerning the chapter on technical considerations.

Dr. K.J. Momose and Dr. D.J. Mikulis, Neuroradiologists at the Massachusetts General Hospital, for their friendly help.

Dr. C.C. Wang and Dr. A.P. Brown of the Department of Radiotherapy at the Massachusetts General Hospital for allowing us to study patients under their care.

List of contributors

Roland Chisin, M.D.
Senior Lecturer in Nuclear Medicine
Hebrew University
Jerusalem, Israel

Nuclear Physician and Otolarygologist
Hadassah University Hospital
91120 Jerusalem, Israel

Richard L. Fabian, M.D.
Associate Professor of Otolaryngology
Harvard Medical School
Boston, Massachusetts, U.S.A.

Director of Head and Neck Services
Massachusetts Eye and Ear Infirmary
243 Charles Street
and
Massachusetts General Hospital
Fruit Street
Boston, Massachusetts 02114, U.S.A.

Max L. Goodman, M.D.
Associate Professor of Pathology
Harvard Medical School
Boston, Massachusetts, U.S.A.

Director of ENT Pathology
Massachusetts Eye and Ear Infirmary
243 Charles Street
Boston, Massachusetts 02114, U.S.A.

Associate Pathologist
Massachusetts General Hospital
Fruit Street
Boston, Massachusetts, 02114, U.S.A.

Michael P. Joseph, M.D.
Assistant Professor of Otolaryngology
Harvard Medical School
Boston, Massachusetts U.S.A.

Assistant Surgeon
Massachusetts Eye and Ear Infirmary
243 Charles Street
Boston, Massachusetts 02114, U.S.A.

Mark Ragozzino, M.D.
previously MR Clinical Fellow
MRI Section
Massachusetts General Hospital
Boston, Massachusetts, U.S.A.

Radiologist
Delaney Radiologists
2212 Delaney Avenue
Wilmington, North Carolina 28403, U.S.A.

Alfred L. Weber, M.D.
Professor of Radiology
Harvard Medical School
Boston, Massachusetts, U.S.A.

Chief of Radiology
Massachusetts Eye and Ear Infirmary
243 Charles Street
Boston, Massachusetts 02114, U.S.A.

Radiologist
Massachusetts General Hospital
Fruit Street
Boston, Massachusetts 02114, U.S.A.

CHAPTER ONE

Introduction

The extracranial head and neck together comprise a region of complex anatomy that challenges imaging techniques. Magnetic Resonance Imaging (MRI), by virtue of its superior soft tissue contrast and its multiplanar capability, displays the normal anatomy and the pathological conditions in great detail. Since surgical treatment is often indicated, MRI provides valuable information for the diagnosis, extent and nature of the various diseases, especially tumors encountered in the head and neck region.

In a chapter entitled 'Technical considerations', we first attempt to give the reader an introduction to this complex imaging technique. We then present, in detail, 35 cases of head and neck diseases, predominantly tumors, that have been imaged by MRI and CT. These cases were selected from 150 patients treated at the Massachusetts Eye and Ear Infirmary (MEEI) and/or the Massachusetts General Hospital (MGH) and who had MRI examinations over the last two years. Most of the CT examinations were performed at the MEEI with a Siemens DR 3 system, and most of the MR scans were carried out at the MGH on a Technicare 0.6 T clinical whole body system using a head coil with a useful aperture of 28 cm (field of view 21 or 26 cm) and a saddle coil used as surface coil for neck imaging. Other images were obtained with a General Electric (Milwaukee) 1.5 T Signa System (Figures 11, 14, 32, 36, 37, 44, 45, 49), a Diasonics (Milpitas California) 0.35 T Imager (Figure 33) and a Philips (Eindhoven, The Netherlands) 1.5 T Gyroscan S15 (Figures 46–48).

The MR images were obtained within a period of three weeks from the date of the CT study. In comparing both imaging modalities, it should be noted that, on some of the images, the section plane is slightly different, e.g. the MR axial section plane is almost truly horizontal.

In every case presentation, we discussed the specific findings of both imaging modalities. We also tried to evaluate the respective indications and comparative advantages and disadvantages of both imaging methods in the diagnosis and tumor staging.

The pathological findings, especially the spread of the tumor (as recognized during surgery) and the pathologic specimen were compared with the radiologic data. An attempt was made to correlate the histological appearance with the CT attenuation values and MRI signal characteristics. Although it is a difficult task to compare signal characteristics with histology, due to the complexity of the relaxation processes within biological tissues, it is the only way to understand some of the imaging features.

In this preliminary effort to correlate MR signal characteristics with the histology, we judged the signal intensity of the tumors on the basis of visual appearance and not of calculated signal intensity values. We also took into consideration that the contrast of an MRI image is very sensitive to the window width and level settings and we were careful not to white out the intermediate tumor signal intensity.

In most of our case presentations the clinical and surgical data were provided by the attending surgeon and, in the majority of cases, the surgery was performed by two MEEI surgeons (Dr Richard L. Fabian and Dr Michael P. Joseph). All of the pathological specimens were reviewed by Dr Max L. Goodman, the MEEI pathologist. This book, therefore, represents an in-depth discussion of the clinical role of MRI in head and neck tumors, with radiologists, surgeons, and a pathologist contributing.

In the chapter that follows the case presentations, we have supplemented the summary of our experience with specific references dealing with MRI strategy of the head and neck region.

Imaging of acoustic neuromas, the temporomandibular joints, and orbital diseases is beyond the scope of this work.

1

CHAPTER TWO

Technical considerations

The interpretation of Magnetic Resonance (MR) images, necessitates a minimum understanding of some basic concepts. Because of the importance of the various MR parameters in image construction, a summary defining the different terms and parameters currently used will be presented first. This summary will be followed by a more detailed overview of MRI physics. Due to the complexity of NMR, only a cursory review is presented. For detailed information, the reader is referred to the articles enumerated in the appended references [1–5].

2.0 Summary

MR images are obtained by exposing the numerous hydrogen nuclei (protons), contained in the large amounts of water found in the human body, to the combined actions of high magnetic fields and radio frequency (RF) waves. The intensity of the MR signal, which ultimately forms the MR image, mainly depends on the density of protons in the tissue examined and, even more, on two other factors; the T_1 and T_2-relaxation times of this tissue. MRI flexibility

allows for a change in the appearance of the images and in the information they contain, by varying the relative contribution of T_1 and T_2 relaxation times. Variation of the relaxation times is obtained by adjusting operator-controlled machine parameters: TR (repetition time), which is the time elapsing between sets of RF pulses; and TE (echo time), which is the time elapsing between the application of the RF pulse and the sampling of the emitted signal or echo (Table 1). The images generated will show tissue contrast, preferentially stemming from differences in T_1 relaxation times (T_1-contrast weighted (CW) images) or preferentially stemming from differences in T_2 relaxation times (T_2-contrast weighted (CW) images) (Table 2).

Furthermore, adjustment of other machine parameters enables imaging in any arbitrary plane (axial, coronal, sagittal, and oblique views) without moving the patient. MRI is characterized by a strong relationship between various factors involving imaging time, field of view, size, slice thickness, spatial resolution, signal-to-noise (S/N) ratio, and image contrast. Therefore, optimal MRI requires a judicious choice of the proper imaging parameters based

Table 1. Pulse sequence parameters and types of contrast (rough guidelines).

Image contrast weighting[a]	TR	TE
T_1	1/2 average T_1,[b] 500 msec	0–20 msec[c]
T_2	⩾ 3× average T_1, 2000 msec	average T_2,[d] 50–120 msec
Proton density	⩾ 3× average T_1, 2000 msec	0–20 msec[c]

[a] The values of TR and TE are dependent upon the tissue pair of interest.
[b] Average of T_1 relaxation times of the tissues of interest.
[c] TE should be as close to zero as possible.
[d] Average of T_2 relaxation times of tissues of interest.

Table 2. MR signal intensity of different tissues with spin echo sequences.

Tissue	Signal intensity[a]	
	T_1-CW	T_2-CW
Fat	High	Intermediate to High
Free water (CSF, edema, cyst, necrosis)	Low	High
Proteinaceous fluid	Intermediate[c]	High
Muscle	Intermediate	Intermediate
Cortical bone, fibrosis	Low	Low
Subacute[b] hemorrhage	High	High *or* Low

[a] Compared to muscle.
[b] More than seven days [14].
[c] Depends in fact on the nature and concentration of the proteins; e.g. inspissated mucous secretions can have high signal intensity.

Technical considerations

on a knowledge of the anatomy of the imaged region and of the abnormality to be evaluated.

2.1 The nuclear magnetic resonance (NMR) phenomenon

NMR refers to the absorption and re-emission of radio frequency (RF) energy by certain nuclei when placed within a strong magnetic field [1].

Medical Diagnostic MRI is almost exclusively proton MR imaging (the hydrogen nucleus consists of one proton). Nuclei that have an odd number of protons or neutrons, or both, possess a property known as spin (precessional motion around an axis, like the Earth's spin about its axis). Due to this spin property, these nuclei (hydrogen protons) have a miniscule amount of intrinsic magnetism known as the magnetic moment.

These protons behave like magnetic dipoles (comparable to a compass needle). They are randomly oriented in the absence of a magnetic field. However, when placed in a magnetic field, they obey the laws of quantum mechanics, and they can be represented as pointing either in the direction of the magnetic field (low energy state) or in the opposite direction to the magnetic field (high energy state) [2–3]. The energy difference created by the protons aligned with/or against the magnetic field is small and is proportional to the magnetic field strength. Transitions from the low to the high energy states can only occur when the energy of an applied RF pulse precisely equals the energy difference between these two states (Figure A); this phenomenon is termed resonance.[1] When the applied RF energy is turned off, the protons return to their equilibrium state, releasing RF energy of exactly the same frequency as the applied RF energy. This RF energy is thus first applied (absorbed) and subsequently re-emitted and this is the detected signal which forms the MR image.

The sum of the magnetic dipoles of the countless protons within the body, placed in a magnetic field, is the bulk magnetization vector, which as a vector

[1] *Resonance exchange of energy* takes place when the frequencies of the radiowave (the applied short burst of RF energy) and the angular frequency of the proton precessional motion, in a certain magnetic field, are exactly the same. This resonance frequency is given by the *Larmor equation: frequency* $= \gamma B_0$; γ is the gyromagnetic ratio (42 Megahertz per Tesla for hydrogen protons); B_0 is the strength of the main magnetic field.

quantity possesses both magnitude and direction. The magnitude of this magnetization vector 'M' is proportional to the strength of the external (main) magnetic field. Its direction is the direction of the external magnetic field (B_0) when it is not disturbed (equilibrium); this direction, by convention, is called the z direction. RF energy at the resonance frequency causes M to point away (tip or flip) from the z axis (Figure B). The strength and duration of the applied RF pulse determines the angle of the tilt of M, i.e.

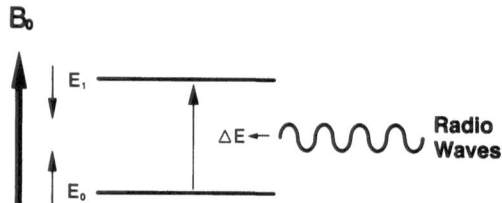

Figure A. *The NMR phenomenon.* Low energy state, E_0, of parallel alignment and high energy state, E_1, of antiparallel alignment of protons with magnetic field, B_0. When exposed to the radiowaves with the resonance energy ($\Delta E = E_1 - E_0$), protons will be promoted to a higher level.

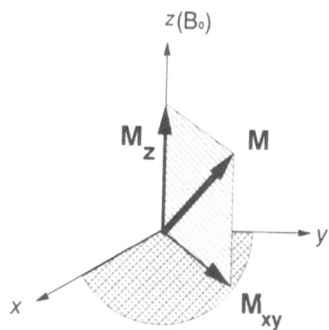

Figure B. *Schematic representation of the vector components of bulk magnetization M*: transverse magnetization M_{xy} in the xy plane, and longitudinal magnetization M_z, in the direction of external magnetic field, B_0.

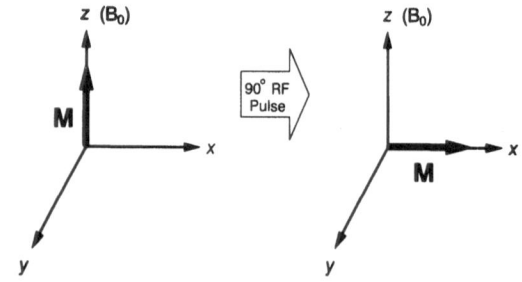

Figure C. *A 90° RF pulse rotates the bulk magnetization vector M from its equilibrium direction along the z axis into the x–y plane.* The z axis is defined as the direction of the external magnetic field B_0.

the pulse angle. The magnetization vector M can be separated into two components: the longitudinal magnetization, M_z, which points in the direction of the external magnetic field, B_0, and the transverse magnetization, M_{xy}, which is always perpendicular to B_0 and therefore lies in the transverse plane (Figure B). Maximum signal (Figure C) is obtained when the magnetization vector is tipped 90 degrees off the z direction (a 90 degree pulse), since only the transverse component of M is detected by the receiver coil.

2.2 Relaxation and magnetic relaxation times

Relaxation is the return of nuclei to their original state after having been disturbed by application of RF energy. Relaxation depends on the chemical and biophysical environment of the protons and is described by the relaxation times T_1 and T_2.

When the magnetization vector has been tilted in the x–y plane by a 90 degree RF pulse, and after the

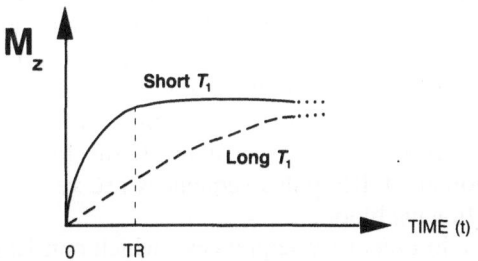

Figure D. *Return to equilibrium of longitudinal magnetization, M_z, (longitudinal relaxation), following a 90° RF pulse.* Longitudinal magnetization vector, M_z, increases exponentially at a rate determined by time constant T_1. Contrast between tissues with different T_1 values but equal proton densities varies from 0 at $t = 0$ or $t = \infty$ to a maximum value when $TR =$ the average of the tissues T_1.

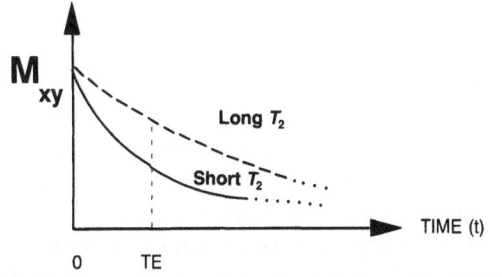

Figure E. *Decay of transverse magnetization, M_{xy}, (transverse relaxation) following a 90° RF pulse.* The signal intensity decays exponentially at a rate determined by time constant T_2. Contrast between two tissues with different values of T_2 and the same proton density varies from 0 at $t = 0$ and $t = \infty$ to a maximum value when $TE =$ average of the tissues T_2.

RF pulse has been turned off, transverse magnetization is at a maximum and longitudinal magnetization is zero. Longitudinal magnetization then gradually recovers toward its equilibrium value, in an exponential manner with a time constant called T_1 (Figure D). Also during this time, transverse magnetization decays exponentially with a time constant called T_2 (Figure E).

By definition, relaxation time T_1 is the time it takes M_z to recover 63% of the longitudinal magnetization lost after the RF pulse $[M_z = M_0 (1 - e^{-t/T_1})]$. T_1, for human tissues, ranges from approximately 250 msec (fat) to more than 2000 msec (water) and depends upon the strength of B_0. Relaxation time T_2 is the time it takes M_{xy} to decrease by 63% in a perfectly uniform magnetic field $[M_{xy} = M_0 (e^{-t/T_2})]$. T_2 for human tissues ranges from 50 msec (muscle) to over 2000 msec (water) and is nearly independent of B_0.

Relaxation T_1 is the result of interaction between protons and the whole environment (spin-lattice relaxation time). T_1 reflects the efficiency with which the environment absorbs the energy released by protons during relaxation. Rapid relaxation or short T_1 occurs when the environment has a high efficiency in absorbing energy, as in the case of fat; long relaxation or long T_1 occurs in the opposite situation, as in pure water [4].

Relaxation T_2 is the result of loss of synchronization between protons (spin–spin relaxation time). This process is characterized by a dephasing of the many different magnetic moments, resulting in decreasing magnitude of the transverse M_{xy} [4]. The tissues in which there are large, fluctuating magnetic fields rapidly lose phase coherence, leading to short T_2. Tissues with smaller fluctuations in the magnetic field have longer T_2 relaxation times, such as liquids and tissues with large amounts of free water, including edema or neoplastic disease.

2.3 Location of magnetic resonance signal

To create an image [5], the grey scale of each point in the image (pixel)[2] is set to be proportional to the intensity of the MR signal emitted from the corresponding volume of tissue (voxel).[2]

[2] *A pixel* is the smallest picture element in a digital image. The grey scale (brightness) of the pixel is related to the MR signal intensity arising from a small volume of tissue called *a voxel*.

Technical considerations

Spatial localization of the magnetized voxel is obtained by varying the magnetic field strength across the subject in a known manner. The variations of the external magnetic field are controlled by small electromagnets called gradient coils, which produce magnetic field gradients. There is a gradient coil for each of the three spatial directions x, y and z. In the 'two-dimensional Fourier transform' technique, selection of an imaging plane (e.g. a transverse section) is done by applying a magnetic field gradient along the z axis, which, in this case, is the long axis of the body.[3]

Once this is done, spatial localization will be obtained in this plane by using field gradients along the x and y directions [5]. These magnetic field gradients change the frequency of the emitted signal. By detecting the frequencies of the emitted signals, we can determine where along one spatial axis (usually the x axis) the signal comes from. This axis is called the frequency encoding direction.

In order to form a complete image (a two-dimensional image), we have to repeat the application of RF pulses many times. The number of repeated applications (phase encoding steps) determines the number of pixels along the other spatial axis, usually the y axis. This process is called phase encoding.

Image quality can be improved by repeating this process many times (using many excitations) and adding up the signal. The signal is proportional to the number of excitations (NEX)[4] while the noise is proportional to the square root of the number of excitations.

2.4 Pulse sequences

The creation of an MR image requires the coordinated turning off and turning on of an RF energy transmitter, three gradient coils, and an RF energy receiver. This series of events is known as the pulse sequence. There is an infinite number of possible pulse sequences, but those in clinical use can be divided into three broad categories: spin echo sequence (SE), gradient echo sequence (GRE), and inversion recovery sequence (IR) [6–7].

Spin echo (SE) is the most frequently used pulse sequence, due to its good image quality and its ability to obtain a large number of two dimensional slices in a relatively short time. It is composed of a 90 degree RF pulse followed by a 180 degree RF pulse. The first RF pulse (90°) produces a free induction decay (FID) signal which is ignored. After the second RF pulse (180°), a second signal is formed, called the spin echo, which is used to generate the image. The time between the 90 degree pulse and the sampling of the signal (spin echo) is called the echo delay time (TE), where $TE/2$ is the time interval between the 90 degree and 180 degree RF pulses.

The spin echo sequence corrects for inhomogeneities in the external field and magnetic field perturbations caused by the patient.

The gradient echo (GRE) sequence consists of an RF pulse, generally with a tip angle less than ninety degrees without a 180 degree RF pulse to produce a spin echo [8]. The GRE sequence does not correct for magnetic field inhomogeneities. Therefore, it is very sensitive for detection of hemorrhage, which appears dark due to the magnetic field inhomogeneity caused by hemoglobin's iron breakdown products. GRE images are also, and for the same reason, markedly degraded in the vicinity of ferromagnetic objects, as well as near air–tissue interfaces. Additionally, GRE pulse sequences are very sensitive to flowing blood.

Inversion recovery sequences,[5] which consist of a 180 degree pulse followed by a 90 degree pulse and a second 180 degree RF pulse, are considered to be useful in examining fat – nonfat tissue interfaces, particularly the orbit or bone marrow [9], but seem to be of a lesser value than the spin echo sequences [10].

2.5 Image contrast

The grey scale of the typical MR image is dependent upon MR signal intensity (SI). Contrast is the difference in signal intensity between tissues.

In CT, the image grey scale is related to the single parameter of X-ray attenuation. There is little flexibility in adjusting CT machine parameters to optimize contrast.

---

[3] A magnetic field gradient can also be applied along the x or the y axis, thus selecting a coronal or a sagittal imaging plane.

[4] The number of excitations refers to the number of times a set of phase encoded gradients is averaged together to calculate the image [5].

[5] *Inversion recovery sequences* are sometimes used to produce heavily T_1-contrast weighted images [7].

The MR signal intensity is strongly dependent upon both tissue characteristics and MRI pulse sequence. Tissue characteristics include proton density (concentration of mobile nuclei), relaxation times T_1 and T_2, flow, and magnetic susceptibility.[6]

MRI pulse sequences can be chosen to preferentially demonstrate differences in selected tissue characteristics. A T_1-contrast weighted (CW) sequence is one which emphasizes differences of T_1 relaxation time between tissues; the image obtained is a T_1-CW image. Similarly, there are proton density-contrast weighted (CW) and T_2-contrast weighted (CW) sequences. Furthermore, there are pulse sequences which emphasize flowing blood and magnetic field variations, such as those occuring in hematoma. Optimization of a pulse sequence, in order to achieve a particular type of contrast weighting (Table 1), requires quantitative knowledge of the characteristics of the tissues to be contrasted (e.g. tumor in muscle or tumor in parotid gland) and has to take into consideration the magnetic field strength and capabilities of the particular MRI instrument being used.

2.6 Signal-to-noise ratio (S/N), spatial resolution and imaging time

MR imaging is a continuous trade-off between signal-to-noise ratio ('image graininess'), spatial resolution, and imaging time. Improved signal-to-noise ratio requires either increased imaging time, decreased spatial resolution, or both. Conversely, improved spatial resolution is 'penalized' by longer imaging time or decreased signal-to-noise ratio ('increased graininess'). Optimizing these three parameters, while maintaining adequate contrast, is the art of MR imaging.

Visual detection of an abnormality depends on the strength of the signal, the contrast between tissues, and the noise within the image. Sources of noise include environmental noise, electronic noise from the imager, and physiological noise (voluntary and involuntary patient motion).

The ratio between the strength of the signal and the intensity of the noise depends upon the strength of the magnetic field[7] and machine parameters, which are selected at the time of imaging. These include, the receiver coil, the number of excitations (NEX), the voxel dimensions, and the exact nature of the pulse sequence.

a) *The receiver coil.* Imaging of the head can be performed using the head coil, which has uniform sensitivity over a relatively large volume. Small anatomic parts, such as the orbits, the temporomandibular joint, or the larynx can be imaged more efficiently and in greater detail, using a receiver coil with smaller sensitive volume and better detection sensitivity (surface coil) [11]. Increased coil sensitivity improves image signal-to-noise ratio and therefore permits reduction in imaging time as fewer excitations (NEX) per phase encoding step are necessary to reach a desired signal-to-noise ratio. The neck images of the Technicare 0.6 T System, shown in our case presentations, were obtained with a saddle coil placed over the neck and thus used as a surface coil.

b) *Number of excitations (NEX).* The S/N ratio can also be improved by increasing the number of excitations. For example, doubling the number of excitations doubles the signal and increases the noise by the square root of two. Therefore, doubling the S/N ratio requires quadrupling the number of excitations, and lengthening the imaging time by four-hundred percent. This method is clearly an inefficient way to improve S/N ratio.

c) *Voxel dimensions.* MR signal is proportional to voxel volume. The voxel volume is equal to the product of slice thickness multiplied by the voxel dimension in the frequency encoding direction, multiplied by the voxel dimension in the phase encoding dimension. Slice thickness is an operator-selected parameter, the choice of which depends upon the clinical problem. Thinner slice thickness, which offers less partial volume artifact, results in decreased S/N ratio. Voxel dimension in the frequency encoded direction is proportional to the field of view (FOV). Voxel dimension in the phase encoding direction is equal to the field of view divided by the

---

[6] *Magnetic susceptibility* expresses the relationship between the magnetic field, induced within a material, and the strength of the applied magnetic field in which the material is placed.

[7] *Magnetic field intensity* is measured in Tesla [1 Tesla (T) = 10.000 Gauss (G); Earth's magnetic field is lower than 1 G] and ranges in the various MRI systems from 0.02 to 2 T.

number of phase encoding steps (usually 128 or 256). Higher spatial resolution, along any axis, results in decreased S/N ratio, which can be compensated for by increasing the NEX or improving receiver detection sensitivity.

d) *The nature of the pulse sequence.* *TR* and *TE* values also affect the S/N ratio [5]. A long *TR* allows the M_z component of M to relax back up its baseline value, allowing a maximum signal to be generated. Since the noise is unchanged, long *TR* values result in better S/N. *TE* is the time delay after the 90 degree RF pulse, during which the signal (echo) rapidly decays before being measured. Consequently, the longer the *TE*, the smaller the signal and the smaller the S/N. However, longer *TR* pulse sequences require longer imaging times. A trade-off between shorter *TR* with more excitations (NEX) and longer *TR* with fewer excitations must be made, taking into account the effects of the pulse sequence on image contrast.

2.7 Image acquisition time

Image acquisition time is given by the following equation:

$$\text{Time (minutes)} = \frac{TR}{(\text{msec})} \times \text{NEX} \times \frac{\text{Number of Phase Encoding}}{\text{Steps} / 60\,000}$$

More than one image can be acquired during the time elapsing between the two sets of RF pulses (*TR*), creating a 'stack' of parallel two-dimensional images. The number of different images or slices, which can be obtained in a given *TR* is equal to *TR*/*TE* + *f* (*f* is a factor depending on the imager), unless

the limit of RF power deposited in the patient is reached (specific absorption rate).

The length of the anatomic region which can be imaged with a single acquisition is equal to the slice thickness, plus interslice spacing, multiplied by the number of slices. If a greater area needs to be imaged, one can either increase the number of acquisitions (which increases imaging time), or increase the slice thickness (which decreases spatial resolution), or increase interslice distance (which increases the chance of missing small abnormalities).

2.8 MR signal characteristics of some tissues

Most extracranial soft tissues have similar proton densities. However, due to great differences in T_1 and T_2 relaxation times, their appearance on MR images will differ one from another, and will therefore produce excellent soft tissue contrast [12]. Muscle, which has an intermediate signal intensity between fat and cortical bone (cortical bone does not emit any signal), and which is seen on all head and neck images, serves as a good reference tissue to assess signal intensity (SI) (Table 2).

Blood flow effects [13]. The appearance of flowing blood on MR images can be highly variable and depends on parameters, such as the exact pulse sequence used, the timing parameters (*TR*, *TE*) of the specific sequences, and even the position of the slice in a 'stack' of slices. All can affect the MR appearance of a vessel. SI can vary from much higher SI (very bright) than stationary tissues to no signal at all (completely black). However, for the most common SE pulse sequences, moving blood typically leaves a signal void, a phenomenon that is most valuable in differentiating blood vessels from lymph nodes or other structures in the neck.

REFERENCES FOR CHAPTER TWO: TECHNICAL CONSIDERATIONS

1. Rosen BR, Brady TJ (1983): Principles of nuclear magnetic resonance for medical application. *Seminars in Nuclear Medicine* 13: 308–318.
2. Andrew ER (1982): Nuclear magnetic resonance imaging. In: Wells PNT (ed.): *Scientific Basis of Medical Imaging*, pp. 212–236. Churchill Livingstone.
3. Koutcher JA, Burt CT (1984): Principles of magnetic resonance. *J. Nucl. Med.* 25: 101–111.
4. Sigal R, Doyon D, Halimi P, Atlan H (1988): *Magnetic Resonance Imaging – Basis for Interpretation*, 102 pp. Berlin-Heidelberg: Springer Verlag.
5. Mink JH, Reicher MA, Crues III JV (1987): Techni-

cal considerations. In: *Magnetic Resonance Imaging of the Knee*, pp. 3–27. New York: Raven Press.

6. Wehrli FW, MacFall JR, Glover GH, et al. (1984): The dependence of nuclear magnetic resonance (NMR) image contrast on intrinsic and pulse sequence timing parameters. *Magnetic Resonance Imaging* 2: 3–16.

7. Perman WH, Hilal SK, Simon HE, Maudsley AA (1984): Contrast manipulating in NMR imaging. *Magnetic Resonance Imaging* 2: 23–32.

8. Mills TC, Ortendahl DA, Hylton NM, Crooks LE, Carlson JW, Kaufman L (1987): Partial flip angle MR imaging. *Radiology* 162: 531–539.

9. Johnson G, Miller DM, MacManus D, et al. (1987): STIR sequences in NMR imaging of the optic nerve. *Neuroradiology* 29: 238–245.

10. Atlas SW, Grossman RI, Hackney DB, et al. (1988): STIR MR imaging of the orbit. *AJR* 151: 1025–1030.

11. Lufkin RB, Hanafee WN (1987): Surface coils in magnetic resonance imaging. *Applied Radiology* Jan. '87: 67–72.

12. Mitchell DG, Burk DL Jr, Vinitski S, Ripkin MD (1987): The biophysical basis of tissue contrast in extracranial MR imaging. *AJR* 149: 831–837.

13. Axel L (1984): Blood effects in magnetic resonance imaging. *AJR* 143: 1157–1166.

14. Gomori JM, Grossman RI (1987): Head and neck hemorrhage. In: Kressel HY (ed.), *Magnetic Resonance Annual 1987*, pp. 71–112. New York: Raven.

CHAPTER THREE

Case presentations

Case 1

ORBITAL METASTASIS OF RENAL CELL CARCINOMA

Clinical presentation

A 50 year old male consulted his ophthalmologist because of a seven week history of swelling of his right eye, with gradual worsening of proptosis, periorbital ecchymosis, and binocular vertical and horizontal diplopia. He also had experienced a significant weight loss over the past six months.

Radiologic findings

The plain films (Caldwell and Base of Skull Projections) showed destruction of the innominate line and the lesser and greater wings of the right sphenoid bone. CT (Figures 1A & C) confirmed the erosion of the greater sphenoid wing and demonstrated a large, enhancing mass located in the superior and lateral orbit, with extension into the anterior and middle cranial fossae, as well as into the temporal fossa extracranially.

MRI (Figures 1B & D) showed an orbital mass of intermediate signal intensity (SI) on T_1- and T_2-contrast weighted (CW) images. This lesion extended posteriorly and superiorly into the anterior and middle cranial fossae, displacing the right temporal lobe posteriorly and the frontal lobe superiorly, without invading the brain substance. It invaded the zygomatic bone and extended laterally into the temporal fossa. The tumor also extended anteriorly into the subcutaneous adipose tissue of the right lateral orbit. There was stretching and displacement of the optic nerve medially with proptosis of the right eye.

Based on the radiologic and clinical findings, the probable diagnosis was that of a metastatic tumor to the right orbit.

Histological findings and treatment

A biopsy of the orbital mass via lateral orbitotomy showed replacement of normal tissues by glandular patterns with irregular arrangements and occasional clusters of clear vacuolated cells, simulating renal cell tubules. The tumor was cellular with scant amounts of fibrous stroma, abundant thin walled vascular channels, and with occasional mitoses. Remaining bone was also identified within the tumor. The histological appearance was considered to be consistent with a metastatic renal cell carcinoma.

A subsequent CT of the chest, the abdomen, and the pelvis showed a large solid left renal mass, bilateral adrenal and hepatic metastases with mediastinal adenopathy. This constellation of abnormal findings was most compatible with a left renal cell carcinoma (Stage IV) with bilateral adrenal, hepatic, chest, and orbital metastases. Because of this systemic spread of the disease, the patient received chemotheraphy with palliative irradiation to the orbit.

Comments

Lesions that destroy bone in the orbit with extension in the intracranial cavity and temporal fossa are often secondary to metastatic disease, especially in patients over the age of fifty. There are, however, no specific features on CT (attenuation values) or MRI (signal characteristics) that differentiate various histological types of lesions.

CT is superior to MRI in the evaluation of bone and calcifications. Small areas of calcification or bone fragments are difficult to demonstrate on MRI, although in this particular case a piece of remaining bone could be identified. Invasion of muscle and dura are better visualized with MRI.

With CT as well as with MRI, coronal projections are mandatory for the assessment of orbital lesions. They define the superoinferior extent of the disease and better demonstrate the roof and floor of the orbits. In addition, the relationship of the tumor to the optic nerve and the displacement of the globe superoinferiorly are best appreciated on the coronal views. MRI and CT are complementary imaging tools for demonstrating destructive orbital lesions of this type [1].

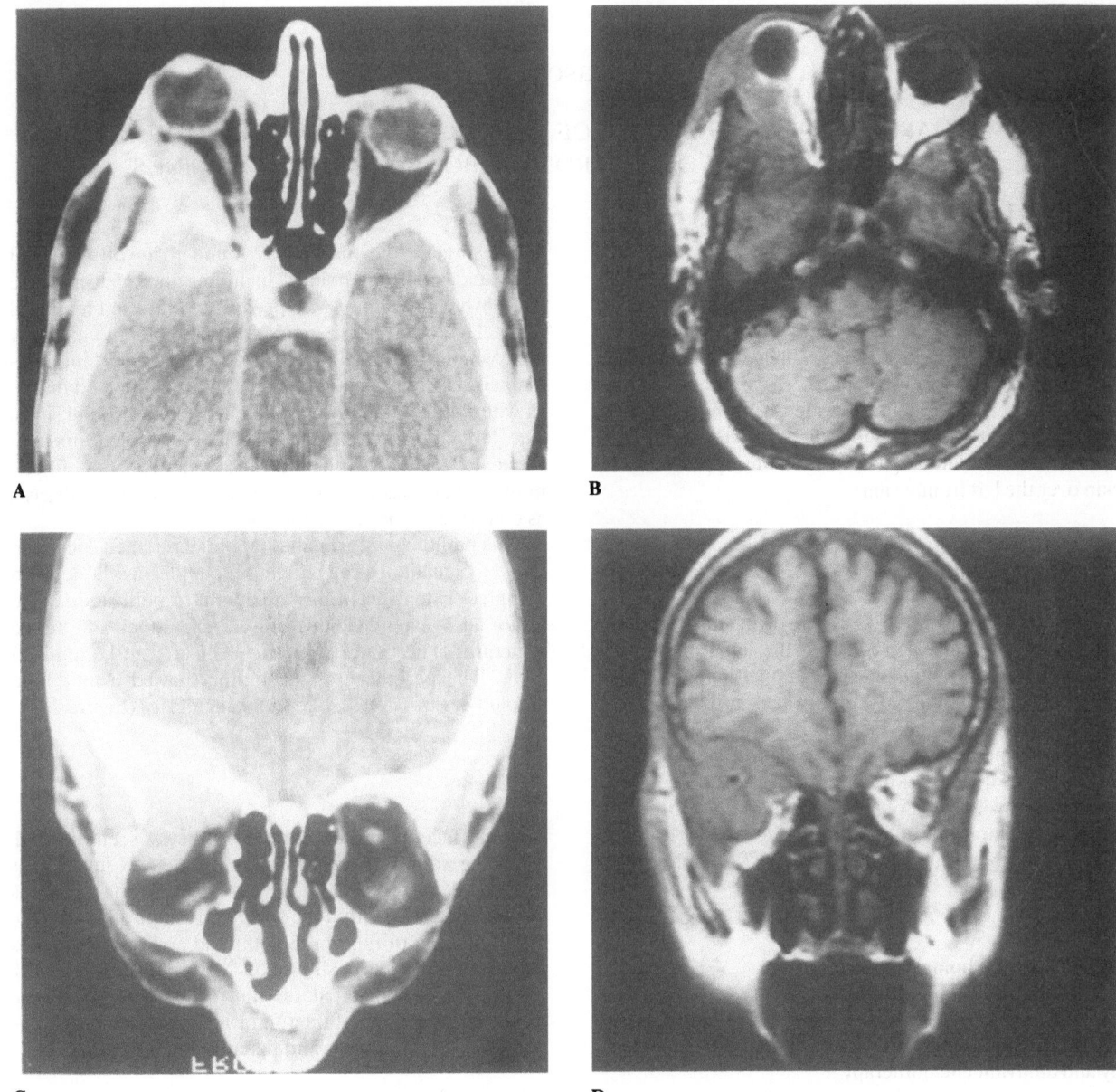

A

B

C

D

Figure 1.(A) *Axial contrast CT section through the mid orbits* demonstrates a homogeneous, well defined mass in the lateral and posterior orbit that extends into the anterior portion of the right middle cranial fossa and into the temporal fossa with consequent lytic destruction of the sphenoid bone. Note proptosis of the globe, obliteration of the lateral rectus muscle, and medial deviation of the optic nerve.
(B) *Comparable axial MRI view* (TR 450/TE 22 − NEX = 4; slice thickness (SLT) = 0.5 cm) shows a mass of intermediate signal intensity (SI), invading orbital fat, deviating optic nerve medially, and causing right proptosis. There is extension anteriorly into the subcutaneous adipose tissue, laterally into the zygomatic bone and posteriorly into the middle cranial fossa with encroachment on the temporal lobe.

(C) *Coronal contrast CT section through the posterior orbits* outlines the mass superiorly with extension through the partially destroyed lesser and greater wings of the sphenoid bone into the adjacent anterior cranial cavity and temporal fossa. Note the medially displaced optic nerve.
(D) *Comparable coronal MR view* (TR 450/TE − 22 NEX = 6; SLT = 0.5 cm). The mass of intermediate SI is centered in the superior lateral aspect of the right orbit extending into the anterior cranial fossa; the dura of the frontal lobe, as evidenced by the continuous dark line is intact but deflected upwards by the lesion. The mass extends laterally through the bony orbit into the temporalis muscle. The optic nerve complex (nerve, veins, artery) is deviated medially. The signal void seen in the center of the lesion corresponds to a remaining piece of destroyed bone.

13

Case 2

SQUAMOUS CELL CARCINOMA OF THE FRONTO–ORBITAL REGION WITH INVASION OF THE ORBIT, FRONTAL BONE AND FRONTAL SINUS

Clinical findings

A 42 year old male complained for over two months of swelling over the left lateral eyebrow. Treatment by intravenous antibiotics reduced the swelling. A biopsy of the remaining mass showed squamous cell carcinoma.

Examination on admission revealed a proptotic left eye with limited lateral and superior gaze and diplopia on upward and left lateral gaze. Tumor was apparent in the skin over the left frontal sinus.

Radiologic findings

A CT study demonstrated a mass involving the left fronto-orbital region with extension into the left frontal sinus, orbit, adjacent intracranial cavity, and left temporal fossa (Figures 2A & C). An MRI, performed in the axial (Figures 2D & E), coronal (Figure 2B), and sagittal projections, confirmed the presence of an aggressive, destructive lesion, along the superior lateral aspect of the left orbit. There was involvement of the left frontal sinus with extension to the dura and invasion of the left temporal fossa. This lesion had intermediate SI on T_1- and T_2-CW images.

Surgical and pathological findings

The treatment plan was to resect the left frontal sinus with orbital exenteration, and to add postoperative radiotherapy and adjuvant chemotherapy.

At surgery, the tumor was found to involve the left orbit and left frontal sinus, including the adjacent dura (from which the tumor was 'peeled'), and the left temporal fossa. The tumor also extended into the pterygomaxillary area where the surgeon felt that macroscopic tumor remained. The left ethmoid air cells showed inflamed mucosa with fluid. No tumor was seen in the right frontal sinus. The large postoperative facial defect was left open in order to facilitate follow-up examination. For fifteen months there has been no evidence of recurrent disease, as confirmed by repeated biopsies.

The pathological examination of the resected specimen showed squamous cell carcinoma replacing bone with complete extension from periosteum to periosteum. The tumor also extended into muscle and other soft tissue structures. The tumor was very cellular with keratinized areas. The periphery of the tumor showed a moderate amount of fibrosis with lymphoid aggregates (Figure 2F).

Comments

The interface of tumor with brain is better seen on MRI. The suggestion of dural invasion, on the MR image, was confirmed at surgery. Likewise, on MRI, the tumor is better delineated within the scalp and temporal fossa. The differentiation of fluid in the ethmoid and frontal sinuses from tumor is clearly shown on MRI as opposed to CT [2]. The intermediate SI on the T_2-CW images of the tumor is a reflection of the tumor histology, which is composed of squamous cells and reactive fibrosis (Figure 2F).

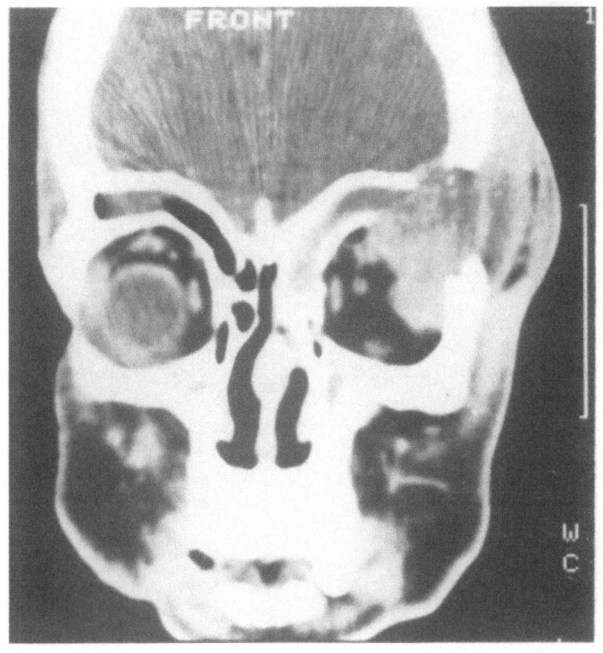

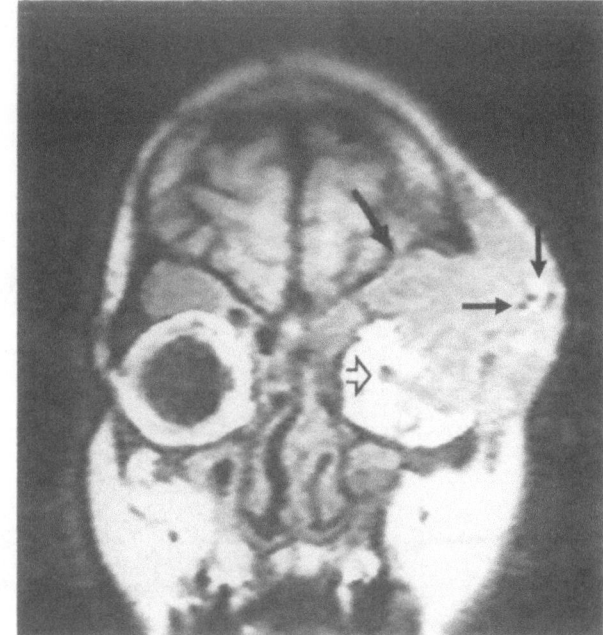

A   B

Figure 2. (A) *Coronal contrast CT section at the level of the crista galli* demonstrates a mass in the scalp with extension into the upper lateral part of the left orbit, supraorbital ethmoid air cell, and intracranial cavity. The mass contains ill defined, low attenuation areas. There is extensive destruction of bone in the fronto-orbital region.
(B) *Coronal MR projection at a similar level (TR 550/TE 21 – NEX = 4; SLT = 0.5 cm).* A large mass centered in the supero-lateral aspect of the orbit of intermediate SI on this T_1-CW image, invades cutaneous and intraorbital fat, encases the superior and lateral recti and abuts the lateral aspect of the optic nerve (open arrow). The tumor destroys the superolateral bony orbit (causing left proptosis) and the inferior aspect of the frontal bone, with invasion of the left frontal sinus and anterior cranial fossa. The material filling the left and right ethmoid sinus displays intermediate SI on this T_1-CW image and high SI on the corresponding T_2-CW image, compatible with proteinaceous fluid (see Figure 2E). There is no evidence of invasion of the brain on this image or on the other T_1 and T_2-CW images. There is a suggestion of dural invasion (arrow). There are small areas of high and low SI within the superficial portion of the mass (small arrows) that correspond to the site of a biopsy performed ten days previously. The high SI can be explained by the local subacute hemorrhage, that resulted from the biopsy.

15

A. Orbital and paraorbital regions

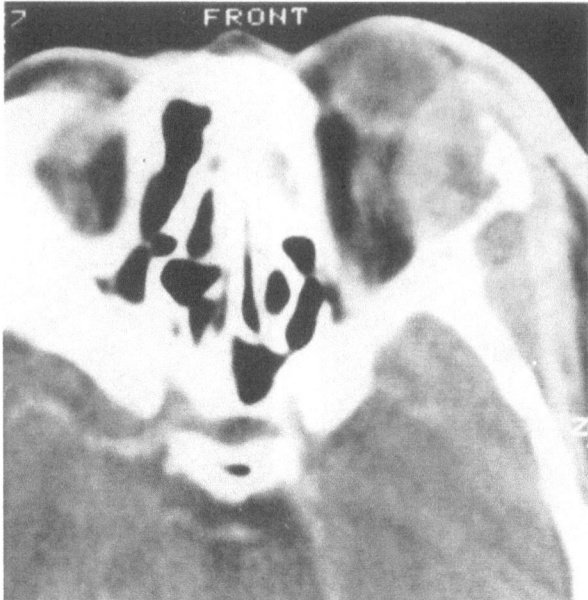

C

Figure 2.(C) *Axial contrast CT section through the mid to upper orbits* reveals tumor in the left temporal fossa and lateral anterior aspect of the left orbit, along with destruction of the lateral wall of the left orbit. Again noted are low attenuation areas within the mass.

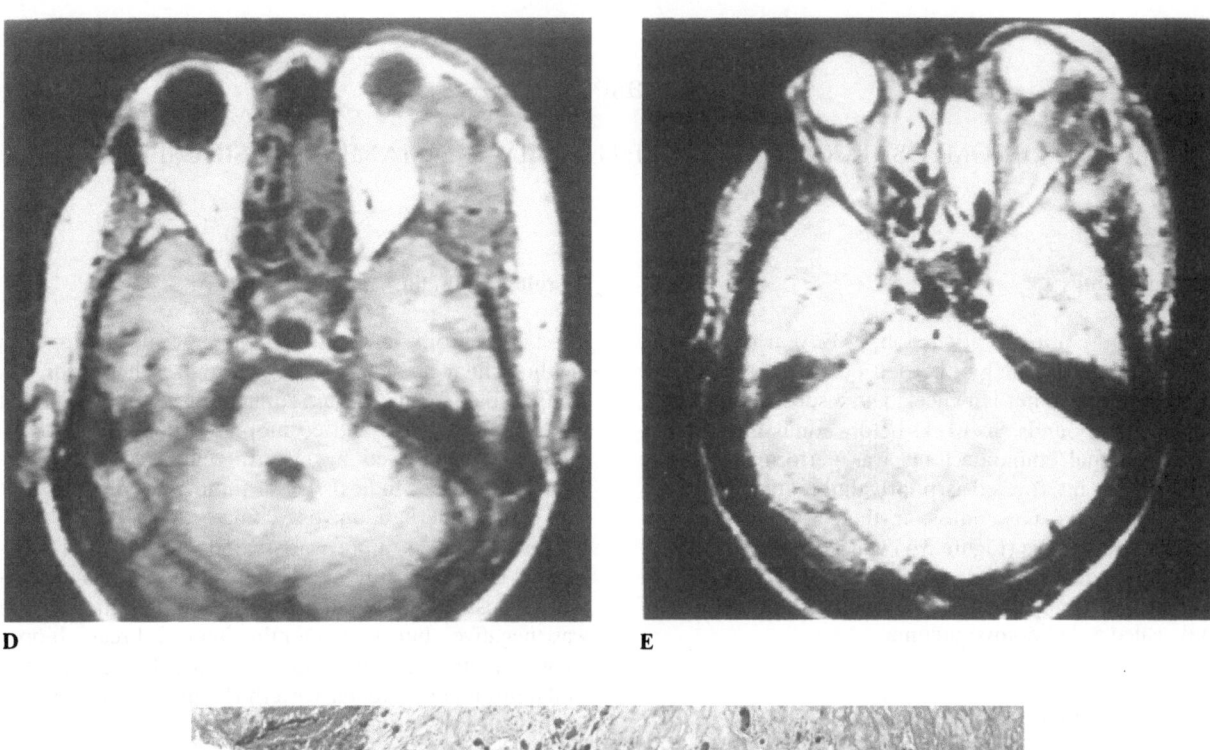

D　　　　　　　　　　　　　　　　　　E

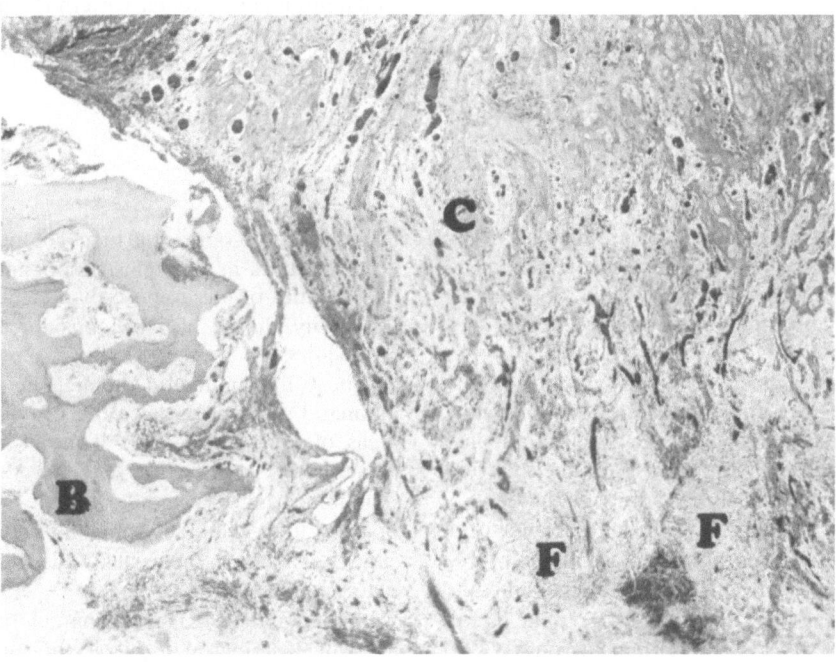

F

Figure 2. (D & E) *Axial MR projections at a comparable level* [(2D) *TR* 500/*TE* 21 − NEX = 4; (2E) *TR* 2000/*TE* 120 − NEX = 2. SLT = 0.5 cm]. The mass of intermediate SI on both images is centered in the superolateral aspect of the left orbit (causing proptosis) destroying the lateral wall of the orbit, as well as invading the intraconal and extraconal fat, subcutaneous tissue, and temporalis muscle. Within the left ethmoid air cells there is substance of intermediate SI on the T_1-CW image (Fig-

ure 2D) and of very high SI on the T_2-CW image (Figure 2E) which is consistent with proteinaceous fluid. Also note the obliteration, by tumor, of the fatty marrow in the greater wing of the left sphenoid bone.
(F) *Photomicrograph from the resected frontal bone* (125×, hematoxylin and eosine stain) shows squamous cell carcinoma (C) replacing bone (B). Note fibrous tissue (F).

B. Paranasal sinuses, including nasal cavities

Case 3

RHABDOMYOSARCOMA OF THE ETHMOID AND MAXILLARY SINUSES

Clinical findings

Three months prior to admission, a 37 year old woman noted pain and swelling of her left eye, decreased vision, and tenderness in her left cheek, and a subsequent weight loss of seven pounds. Six weeks before admission a biopsy via an external ethmoidectomy was performed and the histology was interpreted as 'poorly differentiated invasive adenocarcinoma'. On admission, there was marked chemosis in the left eye (Figure 3A) which was fixed superotemporally with no light perception. There was no palpable cervical adenopathy. A repeat biopsy through the eyelid revealed a rhabdomyosarcoma.

Radiologic findings

Plain films showed soft tissue masses in the left orbit, nasal cavity, ethmoid, maxillary, and sphenoid sinuses with bony destructionn.

A CT study showed a bulky mass extending from the left paranasal sinuses into the infratemporal fossa, the anterior left nasopharynx via the choanal area, and into the left orbit, left frontal sinus, and the anterior intracranial fossa. There was displacement of the optic nerve laterally and of the globe anteriorly and laterally (Figures 3B & F).

MRI, with axial (Figures 3C, D, & E) and coronal (Figure 3G) views demonstrated a large mass at the junction of the medial inferior aspect of the left orbit, the lateral aspect of the left ethmoid air cells, and the superior medial aspect of the left maxillary sinus. The tumor also invaded the left nasopharynx, the dura of the cribriform plate, and the left infratemporal fossa abutting the pterygopalatine fossa, the left frontal sinus and the subcutaneous tissues overlying the frontal bone. The signal intensity (SI) of the mass was low to intermediate on T_1-CW images and intermediate to high on T_2-CW images. There appeared to be no invasion of the brain substance itself. There was marked left orbital proptosis and stretching of the left optic nerve (Figure 3C). The MR findings were consistent with tumor, associated with fluid in the right frontal sinus, with inspissated mucous secretions in the left sphenoid sinus, and with subacute hemorrhagic blood in the left posterior ethmoid air cells [3].

Histological findings and treatment

The biopsy from the orbital region showed a tumor with highly cellular areas and myxoid stroma. The tumor was composed of small cells and some of these cells contained granular cytoplasms and eosinophilic staining suggestive of myoblasts (proved by electron microscopy and immunoperoxidase studies). These findings were consistent with embryonal rhabdomyosarcoma.

This advanced tumor was treated with radiation therapy for six weeks, followed by chemotherapy on an outpatient basis. At this initial stage, the metastatic workup was negative, but four months later a breast biopsy showed metastatic rhabdomyosarcoma. The tissue showed a prominent alveolar pattern (Figure 3H), but resembled the original primary orbital tumor.

The patient died of hypercalcemia seven months after admission.

Comments

Rhabdomyosarcoma is the most common neoplasm of the head and neck in children. Although it occurs in the first two decades of life in more than eighty percent of cases, this entity should also be considered in the older age group [4].

The CT examination defined the tumor mass in the paranasal sinuses and left orbit optimally, along with the areas of bone destruction. The CT attenuation values, however, are nonspecific and therefore, a diagnosis of rhabdomyosarcoma cannot be made based. Moreover, the opacification in the left sphenoid and posterior ethmoid sinuses, as seen on the axial CT views, cannot be differentiated from tumor.

Although the MRI signal characteristics are nonspecific for the histological diagnosis, they do however, separate fluid, retained mucous, and hemorrhage from tumor (Figures 3D & E). Likewise, the optic nerve, in the axial CT view, is poorly separated from the tumor because of its similar attenuation values. MRI quite clearly separates the low SI dura from the intermediate SI tumor.

In this case, MRI was better than CT for demonstrating overall delineation of the tumor extent. It was equivalent to CT for evaluating bone destruction. MRI was also

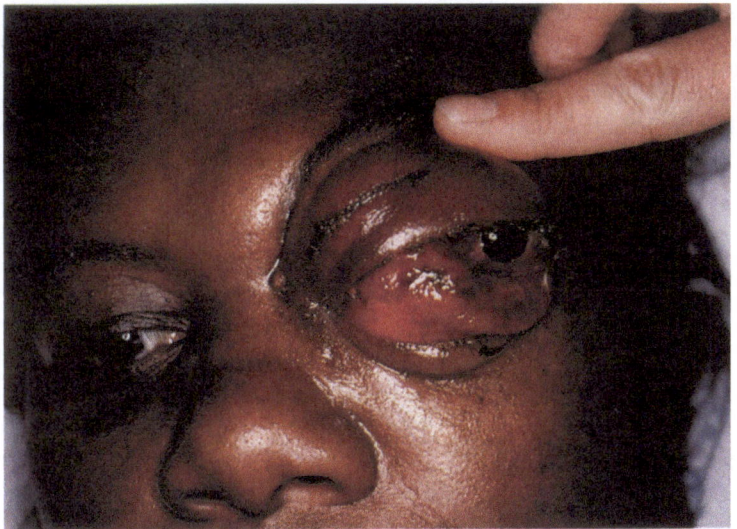

A

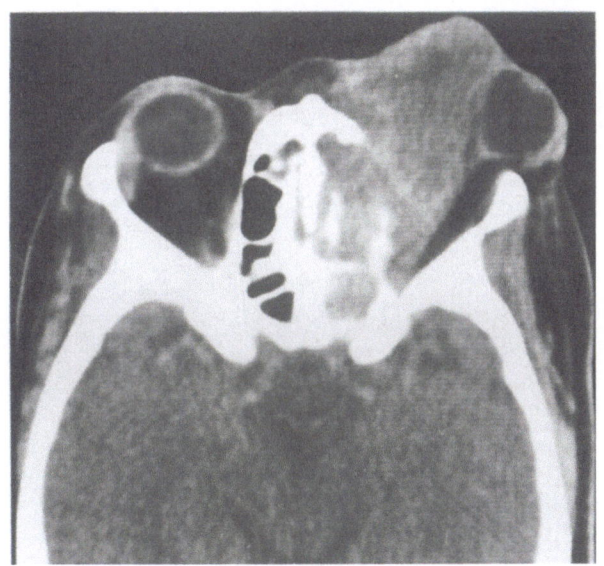

B

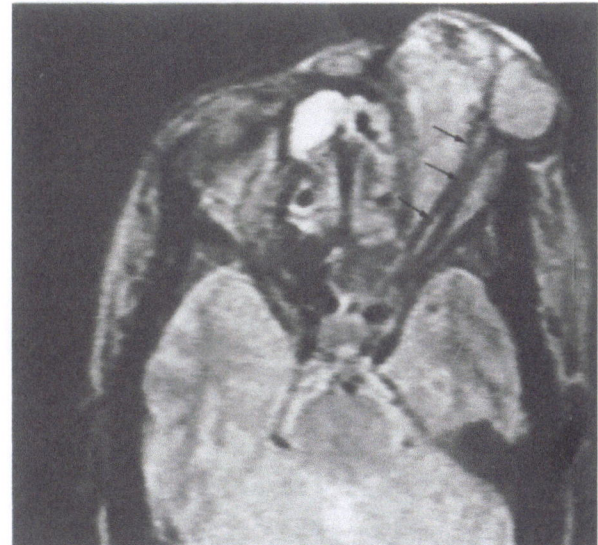

C

Figure 3. (A) *Photograph of the patient on admission* showing severe chemosis and proptosis of the left globe.
(B) *Axial contrast CT section through the mid to upper orbits* reveals a large, homogeneous mass in the central and medial aspect of the left orbit with marked anterior and lateral displacement of the globe which is deformed from extrinsic pressure. There is partial obliteration of the stretched optic nerve which is not defined in its entirety. The tumor extends into the left ethmoid sinus as reflected by increased density in the left ethmoid sinus, along with increased density in the left sphenoid sinus.

There is considerable protrusion of this tumor beyond the anterior confines of the orbit.
(C) *Comparable axial MR view (TR 2000/TE 96 − NEX = 2; SLT = 0.5 cm).* Heterogeneous mass of intermediate to high SI within medial aspect of left orbit resulting in proptosis, deformity of the globe and stretching of optic nerve. The dark line separating tumor from orbital fat represents the periorbita (arrows). The right frontal sinus is filled with substance of high SI consistent with fluid. The middle right and left ethmoid air cells have heterogeneous SI. The posterior right ethmoid cells are normally aerated, as indicated by signal void.

B. Paranasal sinuses, including nasal cavities

useful for suggesting invasion of the dura, but this was not proven by surgery. Meningeal involvement is considered to be the worst prognostic indicator in rhabdomyosarcomas of the head and neck [4].

The relatively high SI of the tumor on T_2-CW images and low to intermediate SI on T_1-CW images reflect the high cellularity of the tumor and the presence of a myxoid stroma (biochemically comparable to a proteinaceous solution).

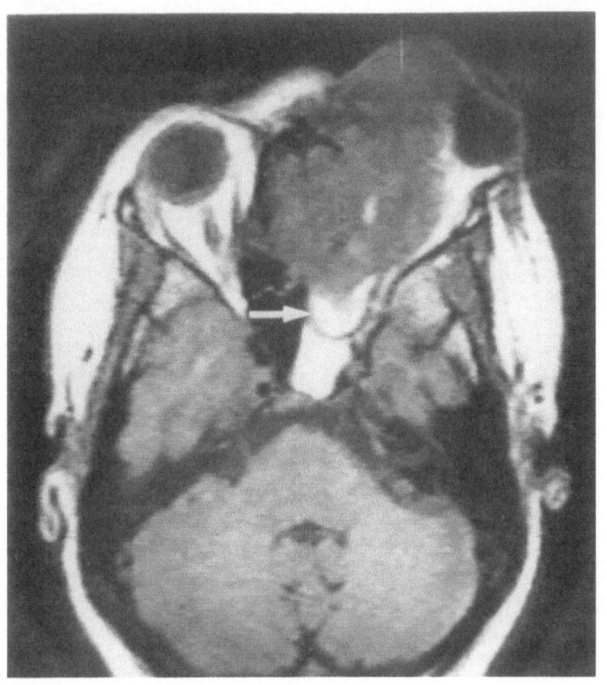

D

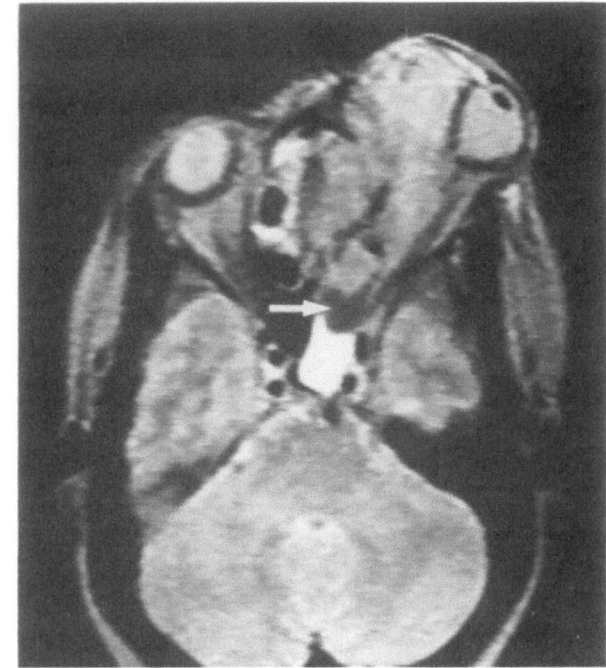

E

Figure 3.(D & E) *Axial MR views at a slightly lower level* [(3D) *TR* 500/*TE* 21 − NEX = 4; (3E) *TR* 2000/*TE* 96 − NEX = 2; SLT = 0.5 cm]. The same mass is seen destroying the lamina papyracea and filling the left ethmoid air cells. Within the anterior and middle right ethmoid air cells, there is substance of intermediate SI on the T_1-CW image (Figure 3D) and of high SI on the T_2-CW image (Fig. 3E) compatible with thickened edematous mucosa or fluid. In the left posterior ethmoid cells there is a substance with very high SI on T_1 CW and low SI on T_2-CW images compatible with subacute hemorrhage (arrows). Within the left sphenoid sinus, there is substance with very high SI on both T_1- and T_2-CW images, consistent with proteinaceous fluid possibly with blood degradation products which would explain the very high SI on the T_1-CW image (Figure 3D). This is most compatible with retained thick mucoid secretions.*

---

* Thyroid colloid cysts also display high SI on both T_1- and T_2-CW images. Their content is comparable to these mucoid secretions.

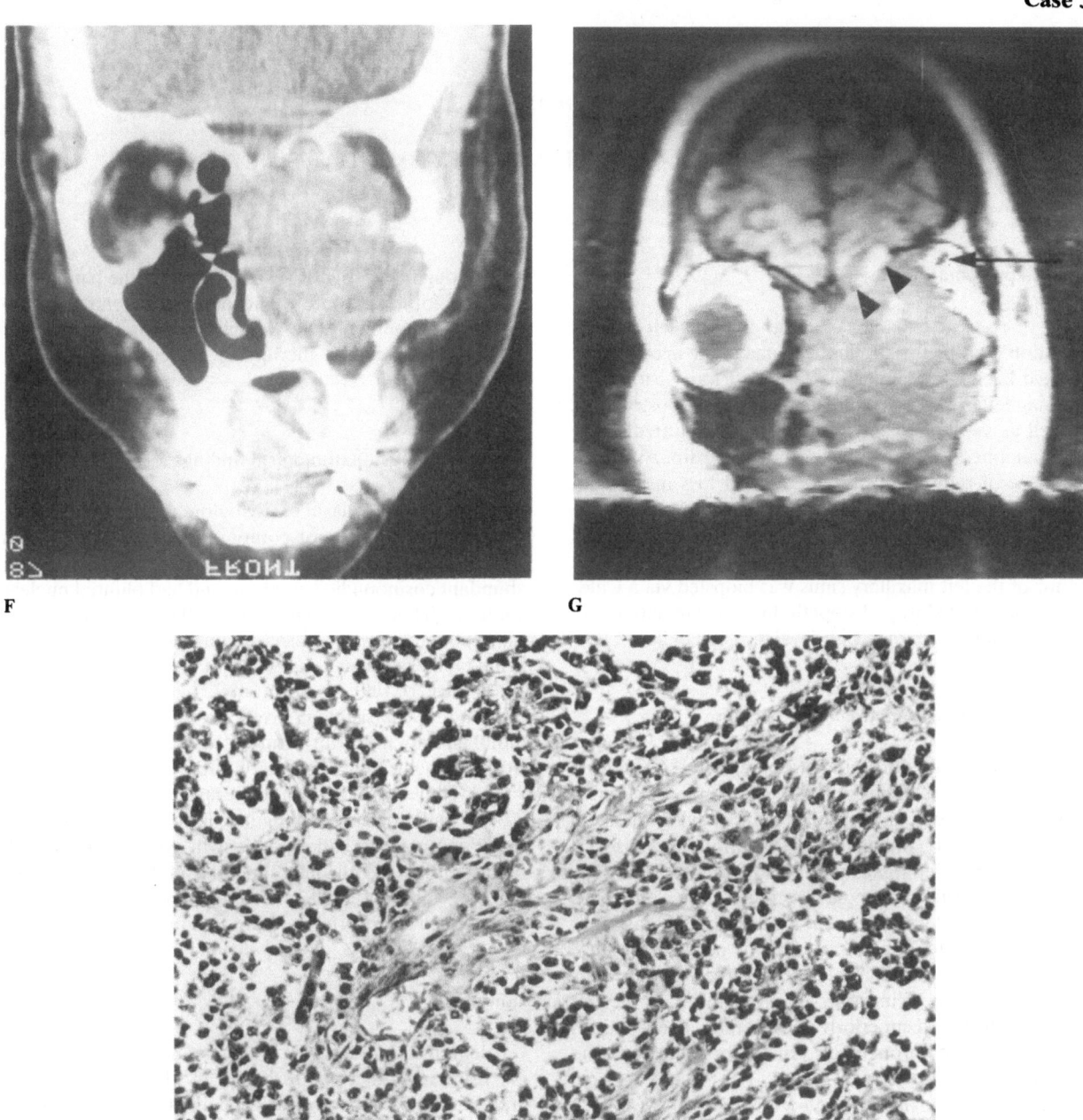

Figure 3. (F) *Coronal contrast CT section through the mid to posterior orbits* demonstrates a non-enhancing, bulky, homogeneous mass that occupies the left nasal cavity, the upper portion of the right nasal cavity, the left ethmoid sinus, and left maxillary antrum with extension to the level of the optic nerve. There is bony erosion of the medial wall of the left antrum, floor and medial wall of the left orbital cavity, as well as the cribriform plate and roof of the ethmoid sinus.
(G) *MR coronal projection (TR 575/TE 21 − NEX = 4; SLT = 0.5 cm)*. The mass, of intermediate SI, fills the left maxillary sinus, left and right ethmoid cells, left nasal cavity, and the medial aspect of the left orbit with lateral displacement of the left optic nerve (arrow). There is destruction of the medial roof of the left orbit and invasion of the cribriform plate. The dark line representing the dura (arrowheads) is not visualized (compare with right side), suggesting invasion. Note signal loss at the lower portion of the image, which is the effect of motion combined with ferromagnetic artifact from dental cavitary filling [5].
(H) *Photomicrograph of rhabdomyosarcoma metastatic to breast* (200×, hematoxylin and eosine stain) shows a cellular tumor with alveolar-like spaces. Note some strap cells.

B. Paranasal sinuses, including nasal cavities

Case 4

LEIOMYOSARCOMA OF THE ANTROETHMOIDAL SINUSES

Clinical presentation

A 37 year old male had an enucleation of his left eye and radiation therapy for a retinoblastoma at the age of three. He had been complaining over the past four years of increasing left cheek discomfort and left nasal obstruction, as well as swelling in the left medial canthal area, along with numbness of the left cheek and upper lip. As a consequence of radiotherapy, he had visual loss in his right eye and only light perception was preserved. On examination, there was a mass in the left nasal cavity. A biopsy revealed only focal chronic inflammation and fibrosis. A tumor of the left maxillary sinus was biopsied via a Caldwell Luc procedure. Histopathologic examination revealed a leiomyosarcoma with focal invasion of bone.

Radiologic findings and treatment planning

An axial and conoral CT study (Figures 4A & C) showed a large tumor mass originating in the left paranasal sinuses (sphenoid, ethmoid, and maxillary sinuses) with extension to the nasal cavity, the left orbit, left infratemporal fossa, left pterygopalatine fossa, and the adjacent nasopharynx. Extensive destruction of bone was found in the left maxillary antrum and left sphenoid sinus with partial erosion of the left pterygoid bone, and adjacent pterygoid plates. The mass was seen adjacent to the left cavernous sinus without evidence of invasion. The prosthesis in the left orbit was displaced superiorly and laterally. There was no tumor extension through the cribriform plate into the anterior cranial cavity.

An MRI with axial (Figure 4B), coronal (Figure 4D), and sagittal views showed a mass of intermediate SI on the T_1-CW images and intermediate to high SI on the T_2-CW images. The extension into the left cavernous sinus (anterior portion) was well depicted on the MR study. The tumor also extended into the left pterygopalatine fossa and encroached upon the cribriform plate with no extra-dural invasion.

Although the prognosis was quite poor, the patient was given radiotherapy before and after an extended maxillectomy. Additionally, he was given chemotherapy after surgery and radiation therapy to prevent distant metastases.

Surgical and histopathological findings

A biopsy from the nasal cavity before any treatment (Figure 4E) showed a tumor composed of spindle cells with abundant myxoid matrix. The spindle cells contained an abundant eosinophilic cytoplasm and had blunted nuclear contours. There were extensions of the tumor into bone. Immunoperoxidase and electron microscopic studies confirmed the leiomyomatous nature of the tumor.

At surgery (left maxillectomy), a necrotic tumor was present in the nasal vault, extending to the roof of the ethmoid and to the cribriform plate, which was removed from below. In this area, the dura did not seem to be invaded. There was no tumor in the sphenoid sinus.

The pathological examination of the specimen showed tumor in the left maxillary sinus with extension to the soft tissues of the face, the lateral nasal wall, floor of the orbit, hard palate (Figure 4F), and to the pterygopalatine fossa. The excised cribriform plate was free of tumor.

Comments

CT demonstrated the mass in the paranasal sinuses and its extension into adjacent areas such as orbits, infratemporal and pterygopalatine fossae. The interface between the cavernous sinus and tumor was poorly demarcated on CT. MR clearly showed the invasion of the left anterior portion of the cavernous sinus, an observation crucial in determining treatment. On CT, the internal jugular vein, internal carotid artery, and the dura could not be separated. However, these structures were delineated on MRI [6].

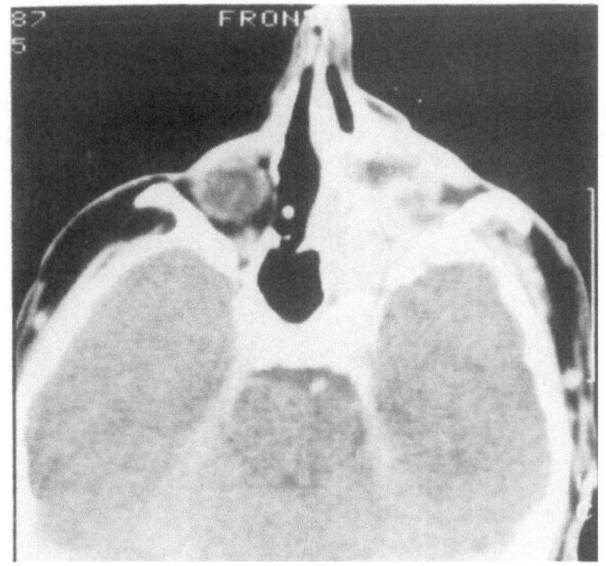

A

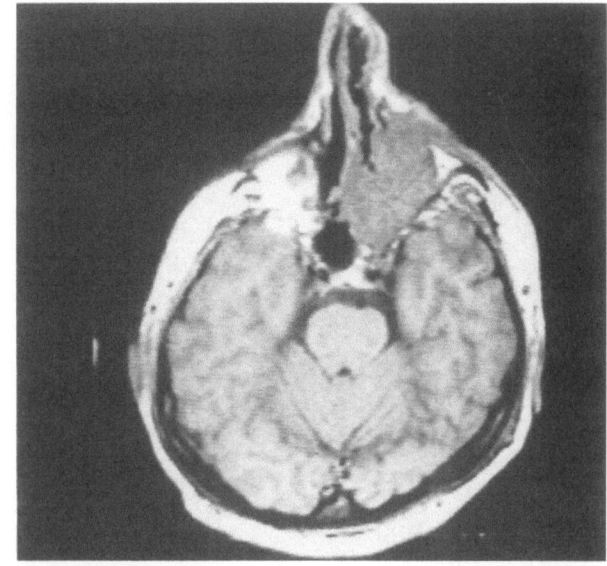

B

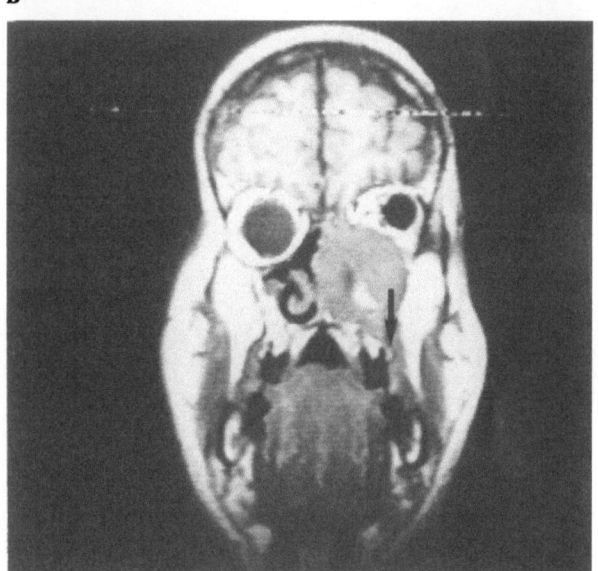

C

D

Figure 4.(A) *Axial contrast CT section through the lower third of both orbits* reveals a tumor mass in the left ethmoid sinus, left sphenoid sinus, and in the adjacent upper nasal cavity with bony erosion of the medial wall of the left orbit and anterior lateral wall of the left sphenoid sinus. The tumor extends into the medial and posterior portion of the left orbit and also extends to, but does not appear to invade, the anterior part of the left cavernous sinus.

(B) *Axial MR projection at comparable level* (*TR* 450/*TE* 22 − NEX = 6; SLT = 0.5 cm). A mass of intermediate SI is demonstrated within inferomedial aspect of the left orbit, superior aspect of left maxillary sinus, left ethmoid and sphenoid sinuses and left nasal cavity, with extension into the anterior left cavernous sinus and subcutaneous fat anteriorly, near the orbital rim.

(C) *Coronal contrast CT section through the mid third of both orbits* reveals a mass in the left nasal cavity, ethmoid sinus, and

maxillary antrum with extension into the inferior portion of the left orbit. This mass has an ill-defined, low attenuation area in the central lower part of the tumor. There is erosion of the medial and lateral wall of the left antrum and of the medial inferior wall of the left orbit.

(D) *Coronal MR projection at a comparable level* (*TR* 450/*TE* 22 − NEX = 8; SLT = 0.5 cm) reveals a mass of intermediate SI filling the left maxillary sinus, left nasal cavity, and left ethmoid air cells. The tumor invades the inferomedial aspect of the orbit, pushing the ocular prosthesis laterally and superiorly. The tumor extends inferiorly into the alveolar ridge (arrow), and possibly into the gingival mucosa. In the central, lower part of the mass, there are areas of high and low SI (also found on T_2-CW images) at the site of the biopsy corresponding to the low attenuation area seen on CT.

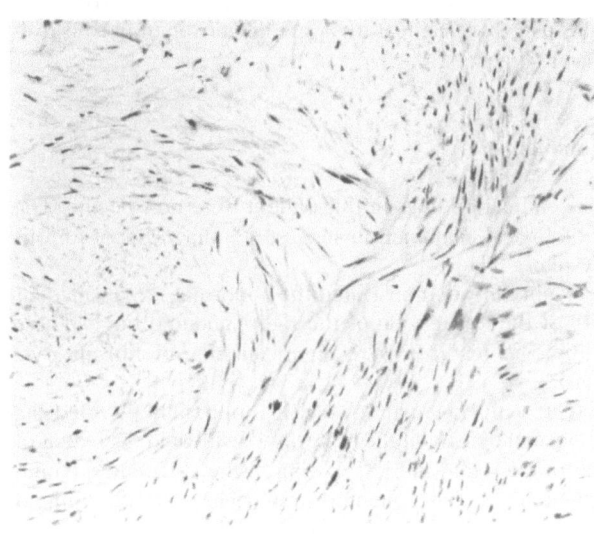

E

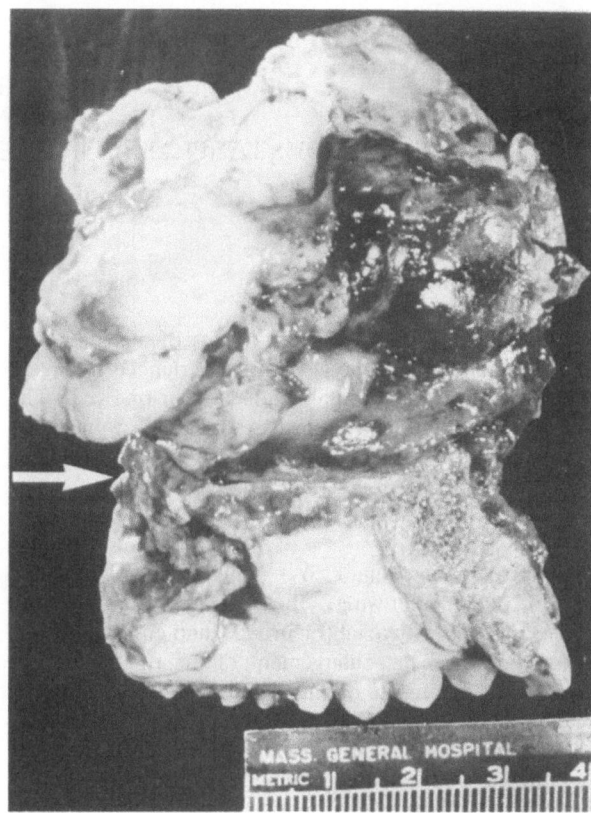

F

Figure 4.(E) *Photomicrograph of biopsy from the nasal cavity* (143×, hematoxylin and eosin stain). A moderately cellular spindle cell tumor with myxoid areas and prominent nuclei is demonstrated. The histologic findings are consistent with leiomyosarcoma.

(F) *Lateral view of resected specimen.* Note polypoid tumor masses extending from maxillary sinus to nasal cavity area with destruction of maxillary bone posteriorly (arrow).

Case 5

FIBROUS DYSPLASIA OF THE SPHENOETHMOIDAL REGION

Clinical presentation

A 24 year old woman had a past history of sius infections and seasonal allergy. She also had experienced recurrent right occipital and bifrontal headaches for one year. The physical and ophthalmological examinations were unremarkable.

Radiologic findings

A Caldwell View (Figure 5A) showed sclerosis and expansion of the lesser wing of the right sphenoid bone.

A CT study with axial (Figure 5B) and coronal projections confirmed the enlargement of the right sphenoid bone, with extension of this sclerotic process into the planum sphenoidale. There was no extraosseous mass.

An MRI, with axial, coronal (Figures 5C & D), and sagittal views revealed enlargement of the right sphenoid bone with replacement of marrow by a lesion of low to intermediate SI on both T_1- and T_2-CW images.

Surgical and pathological findings

A biopsy was carried out via a right external ethmoidectomy. The histological examination showed fibrous tissue and woven bone in an irregular, random distribution. These histological features were diagnostic of fibrous dysplasia (Figure 5E).

Comments

The clinical findings in this patient were nonspecific. The radiological examination suggested a diagnosis of fibrous dysplasia [7].

Plain films demonstrated the abnormal, expansile density of the lesser wing of the right sphenoid bone. These radiologic features were characteristics of fibrous dysplasia.

CT, with bone window setting, optimally revealed the abnormal density of the bone, and delineated the extent of the process into the lesser wing of the sphenoid, planum sphenoidale, right sphenoid sinus, right posterior ethmoid sinus, and the optic canal. The CT appearance was pathognomonic of fibrous dysplasia and is thus the imaging modality of choice.

The low to intermediate signal intensity observed on T_1- and T_2-CW images corresponded to the histological features of the lesion that was composed of fibrous tissue and woven bone [8].

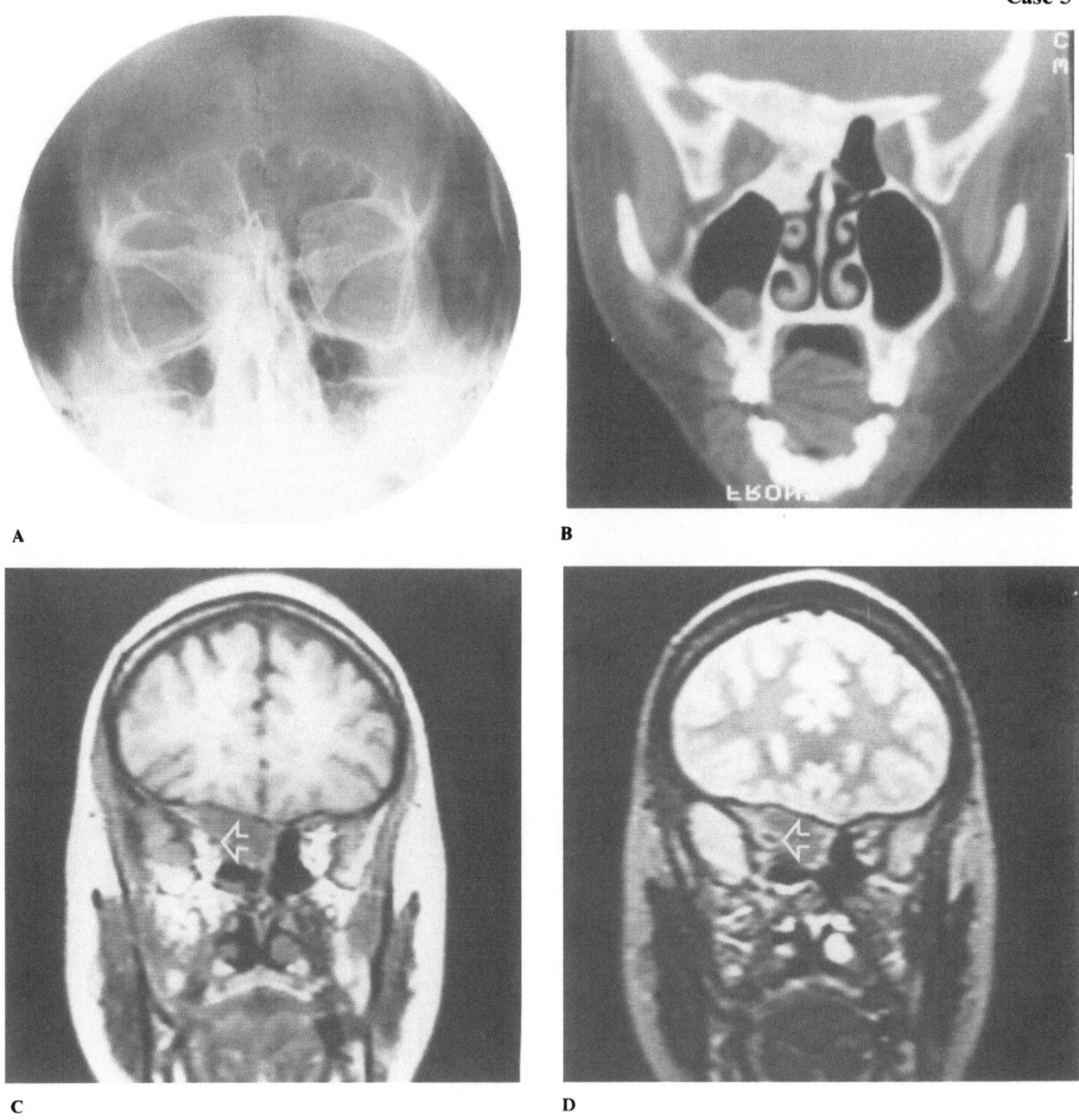

A

B

C

D

Figure 5. (A) *On the Caldwell view,* the right ethmoid cells and the lesser wing of the sphenoid are involved by an expansile and sclerotic lesion.
(B) *A coronal CT section with bone window* setting demonstrates sclerosis and expansion of the right lesser wing of the sphenoid bone with encroachment upon the right sphenoid sinus cavity and extension into the planum sphenoidale.

(C & D) *MRI coronal projections at a comparable level* [(5C) *TR* 400/*TE* 20 − NEX = 6; (5D) *TR* 2000/*TE* 96 − NEX = 2. SLT = 0.5 cm] reveals a mass of intermediate to low SI on the T_1- and T_2-CW images that is centered in the region of the right sphenoid bone, with displacement of the right optic nerve laterally (arrow) and the dura superiorly.

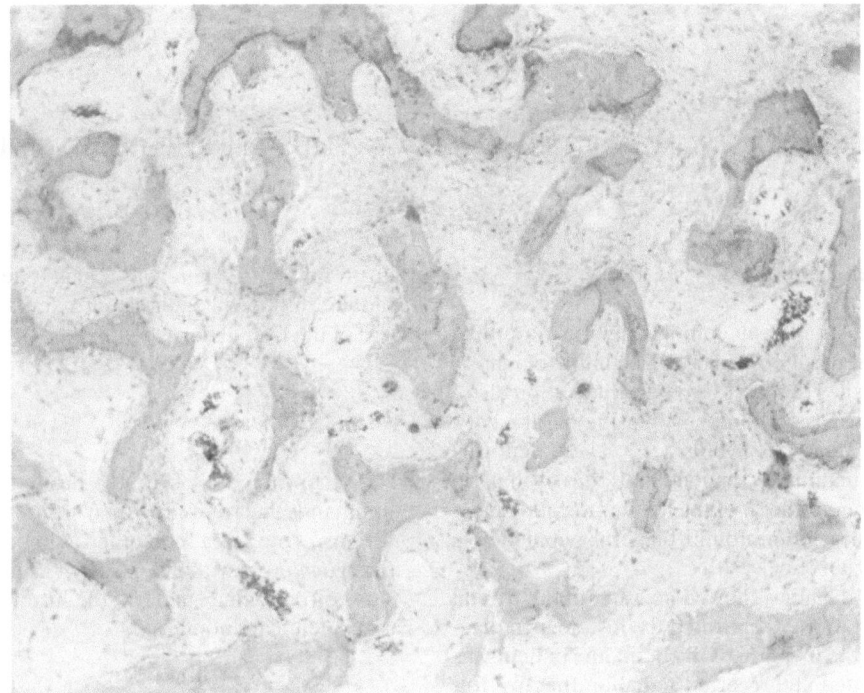

E

Figure 5.(E) *Photomicrograph of bone from the sphenoid area (79×, hematoxylin and eosine stain) shows woven bone and fibrous tissue replacing bone structures in an irregular pattern,* along with prominent vessels. These findings are characteristic of fibrous dysplasia.

Case 6

ADENOCARCINOMA OF THE NASAL CAVITIES AND ETHMOID SINUSES

Clinical presentation

A 24 year old male had been complaining for more than two months of left nasal obstruction. The initial diagnosis was nasal polyposis. He then presented with proptosis of the left eye and a massive tumor within the nasal cavity, and anterior nasopharynx. A biopsy revealed adenocarcinoma. On examination, the patient had some swelling of the left cheek with anesthesia of the left infraorbital nerve, limited left lateral gaze, profound bilateral papilledema, and bilateral VIth nerve palsy.

The radiological studies showed invasion of the frontal lobes and a repeat biopsy confirmed the histological diagnosis. Because of the invasion of the brain, the patient was not surgically treated and received radiation therapy, followed by chemotherapy.

Radiological findings

A contrast CT study with axial and coronal (Figure 6A) sections was performed prior to the second biopsy. The study outlined a large mass in the nasal cavities and ethmoid sinuses, with extension into the frontal lobe and into the medial parts of both maxillary antra. The intracranial tumor incited considerable vasogenic edema.

MRI with coronal (Figures 6B & C), sagittal (Figure 6D) and axial (Figures 6E & F) views, performed two weeks after the second biopsy, showed a large mass of intermediate SI on T_1-CW images, and of high SI on T_2-CW images with marked vasogenic edema of the white matter. The mass completely filled both nasal cavities and ethmoid sinuses, the medial part of the left maxillary sinus, with invasion of the left orbit, cribriform plate and left frontal lobe. There was a mass effect with consequent midline shift of the lateral ventricles, along with compression of the frontal horns.

Histological findings

The second biopsy of the left nasal mass revealed a predominantly necrotic specimen with inflammatory cell infiltrates. One area contained tumor cells with acinar arrangements and solid nests of cells (Figure 6G). Because of this acinar pattern, the histology was interpreted as an adenocarcinoma.

Comments

CT, in the coronal and axial planes, demonstrated the mass in the nasal cavities and paranasal sinuses, as well as its intracranial extension and adjacent edema. CT also defined the bone destruction in great detail, especially with the bone window settings.

MR was equivalent to CT in demonstrating destruction of the cribriform plate and roof of the ethmoid air cells, and invasion of the brain substance. However, it had the advantage of better differentiating tumor from brain edema, and tumor from thickened mucosa and from retained fluid and/or hemorrhage within the paranasal sinuses. MR, also clearly showed invasion of the left medial orbit, as expected, due to the clinical finding of left limited lateral gaze. The intermediate SI on T_1-CW images and high SI on T_2-CW images reflects the histologic observations of large areas of necrosis and inflammatory cells in the tumor.

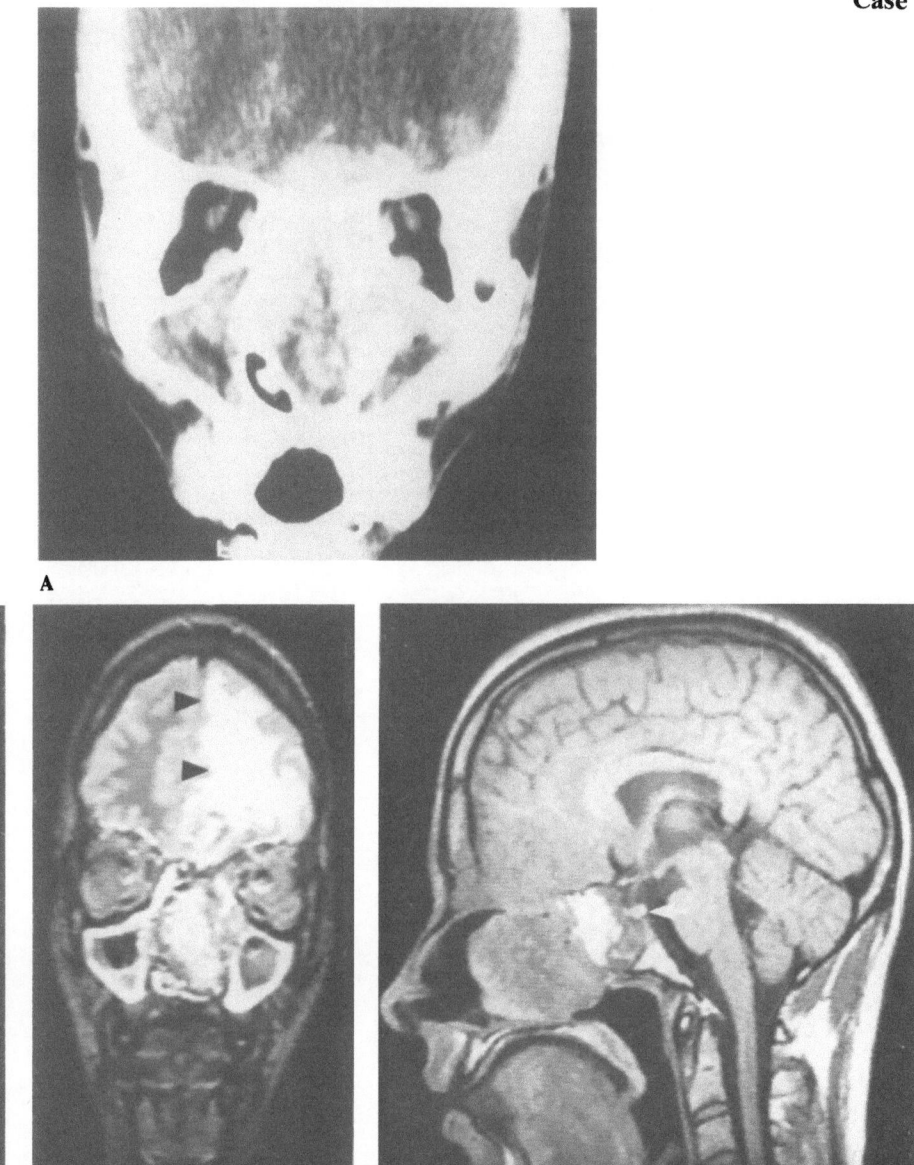

B   **C**   **D**

Figure 6.(A) *Coronal contrast CT section through the posterior third of the orbits* demonstrates a slightly enhancing mass within both nasal cavities and ethmoid sinuses. There is invasion of the posterior cribriform plate and of the roof of the ethmoid sinuses, along with extension of the enhancing mass into the adjacent anterior intracranial cavity. Note the lower attenuation area within the frontal lobes. There is complete opacification of both maxillary antra (the medial parts show enhancing tissue, probably extension of tumor from both nasal cavities; the central and lateral parts show low attenuation areas, probably edema and/or retained secretions rather than tumor).

(B & C) *Comparable coronal MR projections* [(6B) *TR* 500/*TE* 20 − NEX = 4; (6C) *TR* 2000/*TE* 96 − NEX = 2. SLT = 0.5 cm]. A mass of intermediate SI on the T_1-CW image (Figure 6B) and of high SI on the T_2-CW image (Figure 6C), is demonstrated within the nasal cavities and ethmoid sinuses. The mass invades the cribriform plate, inferior aspect of left frontal lobe, and medial aspect of left orbit. There is a large amount of vasogenic edema (arrowheads) throughout the left frontal lobe and a mass effect with midline shift of the ventricles from the left to the right. There is mucosal thickening in both maxillary sinuses with high water content reflected by low SI on T_1-CW images and very high SI on T_2-CW images. The appearance of high SI on the T_1-CW image and low SI on the T_2-CW images within the maxillary sinuses presumably represents mucoid material and/or blood degradation products [9–10].

(D) Sagittal MR projection (*TR* 500/*TE* 20 − NEX = 4; SLT = 0.4 cm). The tumor mass extends superiorly through the cribriform plate and dura into the frontal lobe, and extends anteriorly into the frontal sinus and posteriorly into the sphenoid sinus and the anterior aspect of the sella turcica. The pituitary gland is normal (arrow). On this T_1-CW image there is material of high SI (and low SI on T_2-CW images − not shown) within part of the sphenoid sinus and posterior ethmoid cells, possibly blood degradation products.

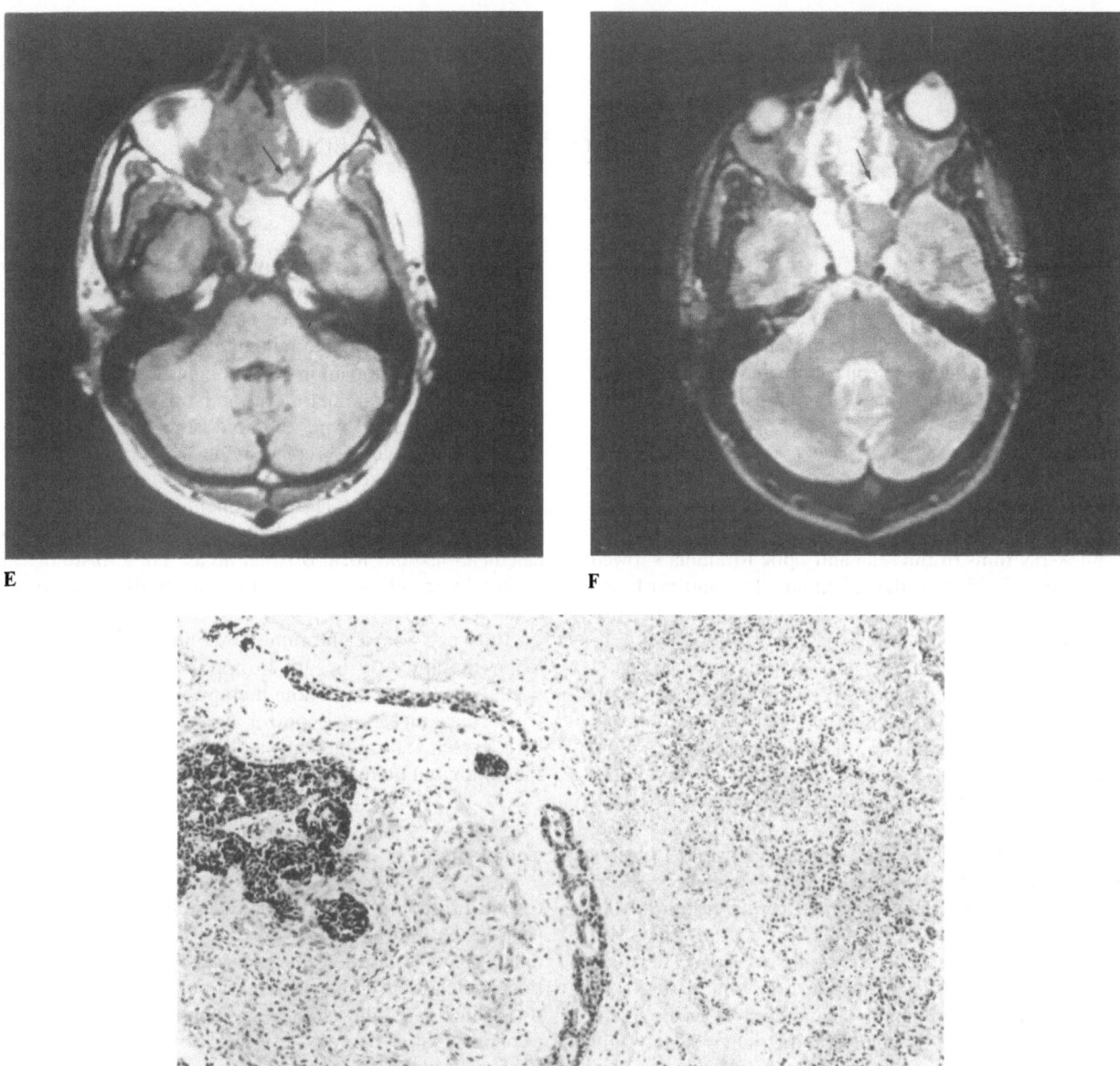

E

F

G

Figure 6.(E & F) *Axial MR projections at the level of the sphenoid sinus* [(6E) *TR* 500/*TE* 20 − NEX = 4; SLT = 0.5 cm; (6F) *TR* 2100/*TE* 120 − NEX = 2. SLT = 0.7 cm]. The mass invades the right retro-orbital fat and causes proptosis. It occupies the anterior, middle and posterior ethmoidal cells on both sides, with destruction of the vomer. In the left lateral posterior ethmoid cells (arrows), there is a substance of intermediate and high SI, respectively on the T_1-CW and the T_2-CW image (Figures 6E & F), consistent with mucous. Within the larger left and the right sphenoid sinus there is material of high SI on the T_1-CW image and of intermediate to low SI on the T_2-CW image, compatible with the presence of blood degradation products. The mucosa of the right sphenoid sinus appears thickened and edematous (low SI on the T_1-CW image and a high SI on the T_2-CW image) without evidence of tumor.
(G) *Photomicrograph of biopsy specimen from the nasal cavity* (125×, hematoxylin and eosin stain) shows adenocarcinoma with extensive necrosis and inflammatory cells.

B. Paranasal sinuses, including nasal cavities

Case 7

CHONDROSARCOMA OF THE SPHENOID SINUS

Clinical presentation

A 40 year old right-handed man had noticed diminishing vision with difficulty reading small print with his right eye for nine months. On several ophthalmologic examinations, he was found to have a right-sided visual field defect.

Radiologic findings

Plain X-ray films of the sella and optic foramina showed dense opacification of the sphenoid sinus and posterior ethmoidal cells, as well as a poorly demarcated optic strut of the right optic foramen.

A CT scan, with axial (Figure 7A) and coronal (Figure 7D) sections, showed a heavily calcified mass, predominantly on the right, involving the sphenoid and ethmoid sinuses, with bulging into the posterior orbits, optic canals, sella, and intracranial cavity at the planum sphenoidale. The tumor calcifications were mottled and showed some confluence. MRI, with axial (Figures 7B & C), coronal (Figure 7E) and sagittal (Figure 7F) projections, verified all of the CT findings described above. Furthermore, MRI showed normal carotid arteries, suggesting that the cavernous sinus was not invaded, and demonstrated the absence of brain invasion. The mass had heterogeneous signal characteristics which were consistent with the presence of calcium and blood degradation products within the tumor on the right side and fluid or tumor, with high water content, on the left side.

Angiography of both the internal and external carotid arteries was normal, confirming the MRI observations.

Surgical and histological findings, and therapeutic considerations

The patient underwent a right transethmoidal biopsy with debulking of the sphenoethmoidal mass and decompression of the right orbit and optic nerve. The central portion of the tumor mass was dense bone surrounded by cartilage-like tumor. At the margins, the tumor was very soft and friable and could be suctioned away. In addition, tumor was clearly removed from the dura of the cavern-

ous sinus, which was not invaded. The tumor that extended above the right ethmoid and sphenoid sinuses was removed by suction. The left side of the sphenoid sinus was also explored and contained mucous. Postoperatively, there was a dramatic improvement in his vision.

Histological examination of the biopsy specimen from the right sphenoid and ethmoid sinuses (Figure 7G) showed cartilaginous replacement of bone and sinus cavity by immature cartilage cells with areas of ossification and calcification. The components were hyaline cartilage, myxoid cartilage, and degenerating cartilage with calcifications and focal ossified areas. These histological features were characteristic of Grade II/III chondrosarcoma.

Total excision of the tumor was not possible. Proton beam therapy was begun. Proton beams provide high spatial resolution radiation therapy of deep structures, which maximizes local control and minimizes morbidity [11]. Repeat CT studies showed increased calcification of the tumor, but no further expansion.

Comments

Chondrosarcoma of the paranasal sinuses is an uncommon lesion, but should be considered in the differential diagnosis of a calcified mass, especially if bone destruction is identified. Other lesions to be considered include osteogenic sarcoma, chordoma, meningioma, osteoblastoma, and fibro-osseous lesions (ossifying fibroma and fibrous dysplasia).

Neither CT nor MR could preclude the need for a surgical biopsy prior to treatment. Both modalities were valuable for staging.

In this case, CT proved to be superior for demonstrating bone erosion and matrix calcification. There are no distinct features of the CT appearance of chondrosarcomas, which permit differentiation from other calcified destructive lesions, such as chordomas [12].

Chordomas are less common in the paranasal sinuses, and more common in the area of the clivus and sella, where notochordal remnants, from which they arise, are located.

MR was less sensitive than CT in the demonstration of calcification, characterized by a signal void. MR was

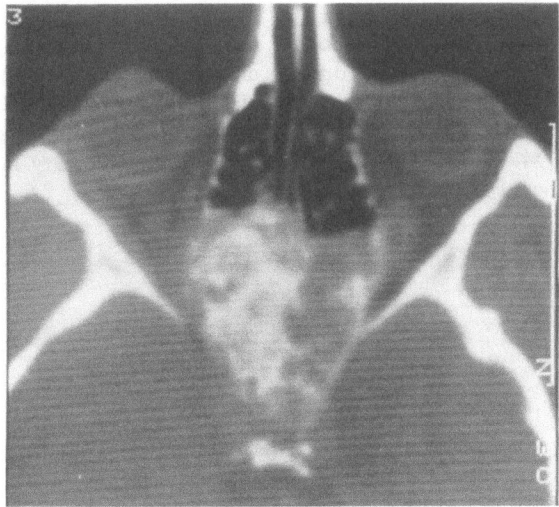

A

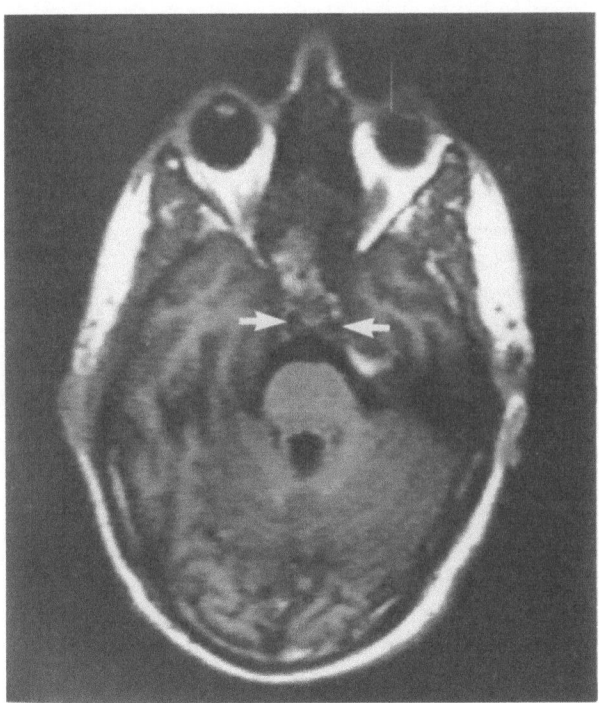

B

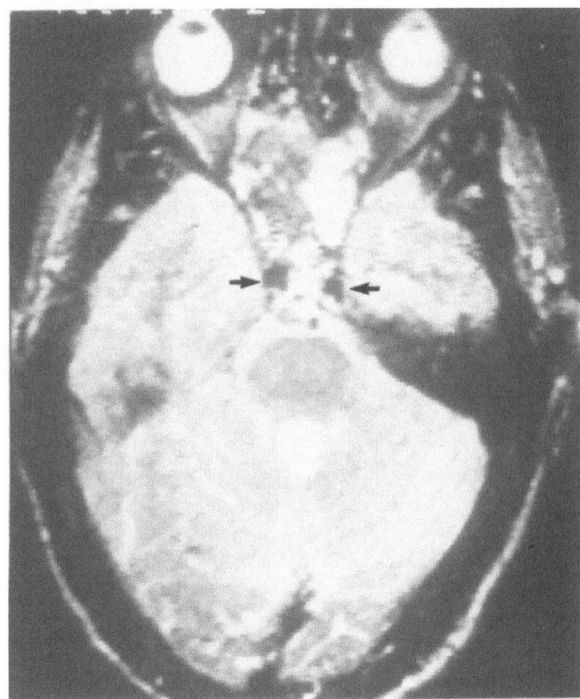

C

Figure 7. (A) *Axial CT section with bone window setting at the level of mid orbits* reveals a densely calcified mass in the sphenoid sinus and posterior ethmoid air cells, bulging into the medial posterior third of both orbits. The mass also bulges into the superior orbital fissures and anterior sellar cavity. Note the slightly irregular border of this mass on the right.
(B & C) *Axial MR projections at comparable level* [(7B) *Inversion recovery pulse sequence* (IR)* − *TR* 1500/T_1 450/*TE* 20 − NEX = 2. (7C) *Spin echo pulse sequence* (SE) − *TR* 2000/*TE* 120 − NEX = 2. STL = 0.7 cm]. There is a midline mass with

heterogeneous signal characteristics filling posterior ethmoid air cells and sphenoid sinus. Although the mass abuts the cavernous sinus, it is uncertain whether the cavernous sinus is invaded. However, the carotid arteries (arrows) are patent without evidence of encasement to suggest cavernous invasion. The left side of the mass has a low SI on the T_1-CW image (Figure 7B) and intermediate to high SI on the T_2-CW image (Figure 7C), consistent with fluid or soft tissue with high water content. The right side of the mass has heterogeneous SI, with predominantly low SI on both T_1- and T_2-CW images, interspersed with small areas of high SI. The findings are compatible with a calcified soft tissue mass.

* (IR) is used here to generate a T_1-CW image.

B. Paranasal sinuses, including nasal cavities

superior to CT in showing the relationship of the tumor mass to the adjacent frontal lobe and carotid arteries, due to its superior soft tissue contrast and its multiplanar capability.

Although the heterogeneity of MR signal characteristics suggested a complex histological composition of the tumor (hyaline myxoid degenerative cartilage, ossified areas, bone marrow), the histology underlying these SI changes could not be precisely determined.

In addition, information from both CT and MR seems to be complementary in planning proton beam therapy [13].

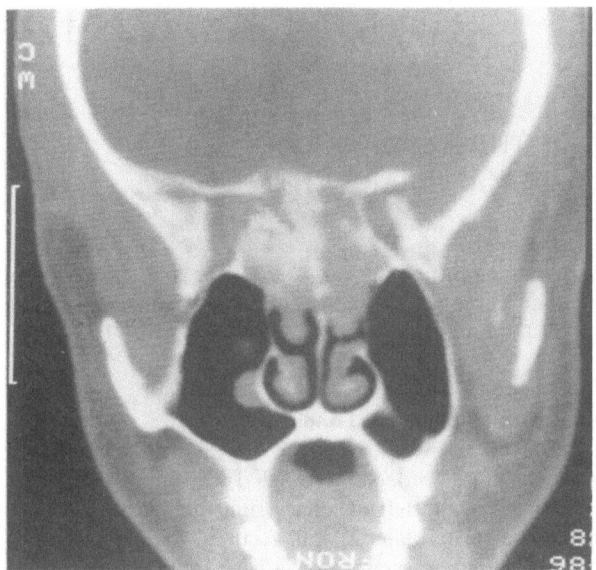

D

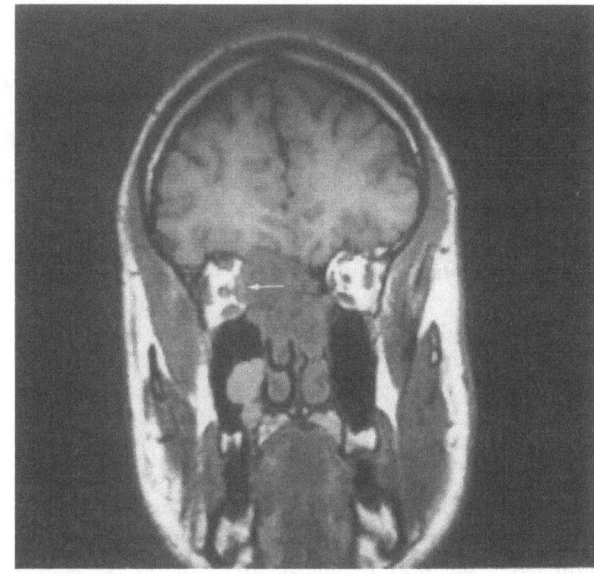

E

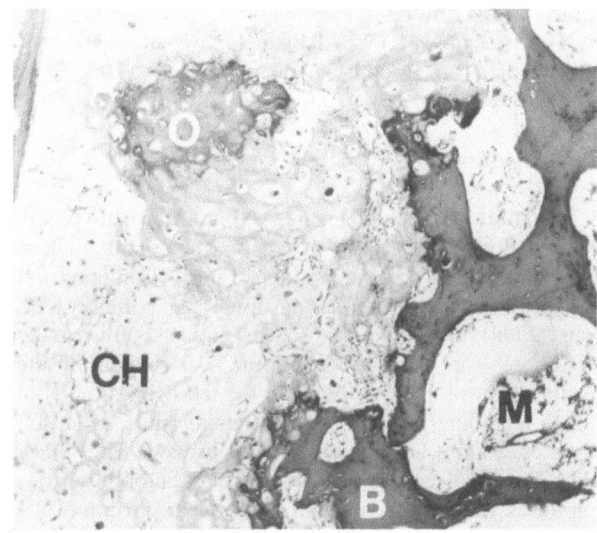

F

G

Figure 7. (D) *Coronal CT section with bone window setting through the level of mid sphenoid sinus and posterior orbits* shows a partially calcified mass extending into the upper third of both nasal cavities. There is elevation of the planum sphenoidale on the right, as well as irregularity and partial loss of the medial posterior wall of the right orbit. Note also a retention cyst in the lower medial right antrum.

(E) *Coronal MR projection at similar level (TR 500/TE 20 − NEX = 4; SLT = 0.5 cm).* A midline mass of intermediate SI invades the ethmoid cells bilaterally, and the superior part of the nasal cavity, obliterating the upper middle turbinates. The tumor invades the medial aspect of the right orbit with displacement of the medial rectus muscle (arrow). The cribriform plate is invaded (mainly on the right side), with superior deviation of the dura, without invasion of the right frontal lobe. Two sharply defined masses within the right maxillary sinus exhibit fairly high SI on

T_1-CW (and high SI on T_2-CW images). They are consistent with mucous retention cysts.

(F) *Right parasagittal MR projection (TR 500/TE 20 NEX = 4; SLT = 0.5 cm).* A mass of heterogeneous SI is located in the sphenoid sinus and posterior ethmoid cells, with extension to the middle ethmoid cells, posterior nasal cavity, superior nasopharynx, tuberculum sellae, and planum sphenoidale. The mass elevates the dura and frontal lobe without invasion of brain substance. The irregular, high SI areas within the mass are compatible with retained thick mucous secretions and/or blood degradation products.

(G) *Photomicrograph of biopsy from sphenoid sinus (12×, hematoxylin and eosin stain)* shows replacement of bone (B) by chondrosarcoma (CH) with focal areas of ossification (O). Bone marrow spaces (M).

39

Case 8

SQUAMOUS CELL CARCINOMA OF THE NASOPHARYNX, PARANASOPHARYNGEAL SPACE, AND MAXILLARY ANTRUM

Clinical presentation

A 49 year old woman had been treated for bilateral serous otitis media with insertion of ventilating tubes one and one-half years prior to admission. She later complained of left nasal congestion and left facial pain, along with numbness in her left cheek and trismus. Examination upon admission revealed fullness of her left cheek with decreased sensation, and a firm, 1.5 cm left submandibular lymph node. Soon after, she developed a complete VIth nerve palsy. A radiologic investigation revealed a mass extending from the left maxillary sinus to the base of the skull. A left transantral biopsy was performed and revealed poorly differentiated squamous cell carcinoma.

The patient was treated by palliative chemotherapy, and she died three months later.

Radiologic findings

A CT study with axial (Figure 8A) and coronal (Figure 8C) sections showed an extensive, mixed attenuation tumor that involved the maxillary antra, infratemporal and pterygopalatine fossae, nasopharynx, paranasopharyngeal and retropharyngeal spaces, and cavernous sinuses. There was extensive lytic bone destruction of the maxillary antra, posterior wall of the left orbit, pterygoid bones including plates, clivus, sphenoid sinus, sella, left optic canal, and left anterior clinoid process. The tumor mass also involved the middle cranial fossa, both petrous pyramids, the hard palate, and the alveolar portion of the left maxilla.

An MRI with axial (Figure 8B), coronal (Figures 8D & E), and sagittal views demonstrated a large, midline, destructive process extending from the hard palate to the sella turcica, and involving the left maxillary sinus, alveolar ridge, and both petrous apices. The tumor invaded the cavernous sinus and encased both carotid arteries and in-

vaded both infratemporal fossae. The mass had intermediate SI on T_1-CW images and intermediate to high SI on T_2-CW images.

Surgical and histological findings

A Caldwell Luc procedure revealed clear mucoid liquid in the center of the left maxillary sinus and a friable mass along the posterolateral wall. A tissue biopsy from the maxillary sinus mass showed a very cellular tumor with massive necrosis, composed of ovoid cells in nests and sheets, with areas of squamous differentiation (Figure 8F). The tumor was ulcerated and focally involved the mucosa, while other portions of the mucosa were inflamed, but not invaded by tumor (Figure 8G). The tumor invaded the sinus mucosa, nerves, perivascular areas, and bone. The tumor morphology was consistent with a poorly differentiated squamous cell carcinoma.

Comments

The CT demonstrated the areas of bone destruction in detail. The boundaries of the tumor were difficult to define in the paranasopharyngeal spaces and infratemporal fossae.

CT poorly visualized the carotid arteries. However, on MR, the encasement of the petrous portion of the internal carotid arteries by tumor was well depicted. MR was superior to CT in demonstrating tumor invasion of the cavernous sinuses and sella turcica, as well as the relationship of the tumor to the cavernous portions of the carotid arteries, and the tumor extension into the nasopharynx, paranasopharyngeal and retropharyngeal spaces.

The intermediate to high SI on the T_2-CW images is consistent with the tumor necrosis illustrated on the histologic section.

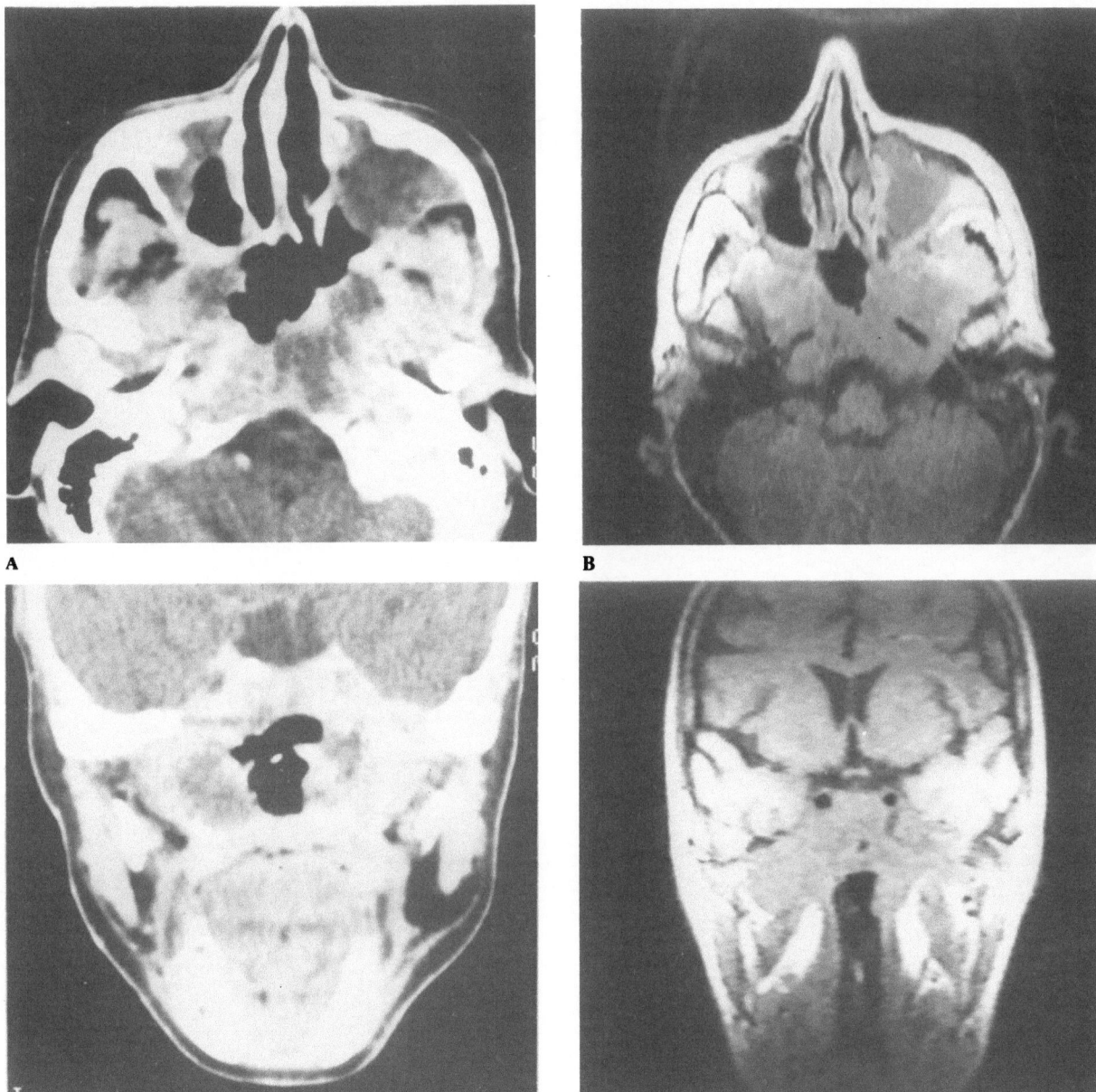

Figure 8.(A) *Axial contrast CT section through the mid portion of both maxillary antra* reveals a mass of mixed attenuation (isodense with muscle along with areas of low attenuation) in both maxillary antra, the paranasopharyngeal spaces, infratemporal and pterygopalatine fossae, and in the retropharyngeal space. This tumor causes extensive destruction of the lateral and posterior walls of the left antrum, the medial third of the posterior wall of the right antrum, and the pterygoid bones and plates.
(B) *Axial MR projection at a comparable level* (*TR* 500/*TE* 21 − NEX = 6; SLT = 0.5 cm). A mass of intermediate SI is demonstrated, centered within the nasopharynx, destroying the clivus and petrous apices, encasing both carotid arteries, and invading both infratemporal and pterygopalatine fossae. The left maxillary sinus is filled with material of relatively low SI on this T_1-

CW image (and high SI on this T_2-CW images − not illustrated) compatible with fluid.
(C) *Coronal contrast CT section through the sellar area* reveals destruction of the sella, the clivus, and floor of the middle cranial fossa bilaterally. There is a mass in the nasopharynx and paranasopharyngeal spaces with extension into the middle cranial fossa. There are low attenuation areas within this isodense mass, compatible with necrosis.
(D) *Comparable coronal MR projection* (*TR* 500/*TE* 21 − NEX = 4; SLT = 0.5 cm). The mass invades the sphenoid sinus, clivus, sella turcica, cavernous sinuses and infratemporal fossae bilaterally. The dura of the medial aspect of the left middle cranial fossa is not well visualized suggesting dural invasion; however, the temporal lobes are not invaded. The tumor encases both carotid arteries.

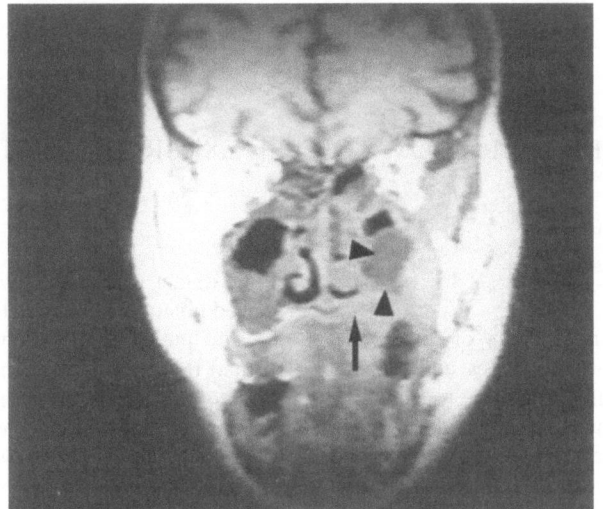

E

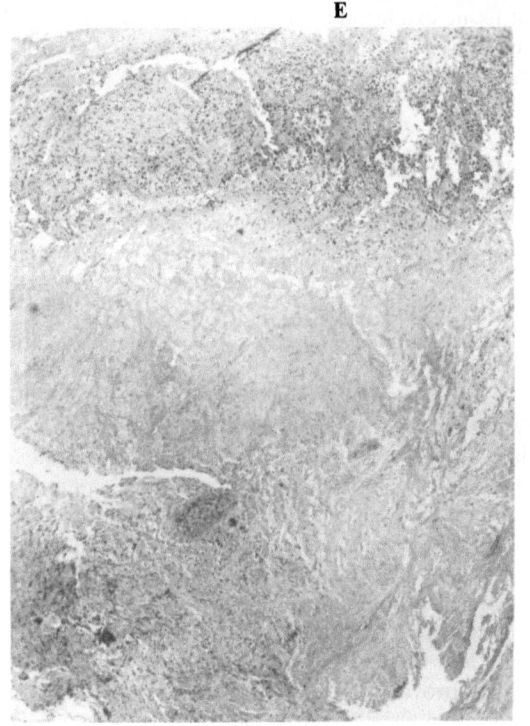

F

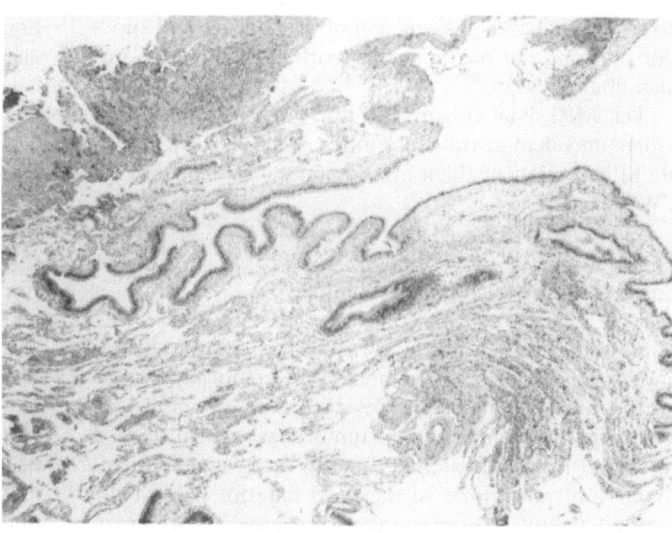

G

Figure 8. (E) *Coronal MR projection through posterior third of orbits (TR 500/TE 21 − NEX = 4; SLT = 0.5 cm).* There is a mass of intermediate SI seen along the medial, inferior, and lateral aspects of the left maxillary sinus, with extension inferiorly to the hard plate and alveolar ridge. The marrow of these structures is obliterated (arrow). The mass spreads along the lateral wall of the left orbit and left maxillary sinus. The substance of low SI on this T_1-CW image (high SI on T_2-CW images not illustrated) partially filling the left maxillary sinus represents fluid (arrowheads). The rim of low to intermediate SI on T_1-CW images (high SI on T_2-CW images not shown) outlining the right maxillary sinus is consistent with thickened edematous mucosa.

(F) *Photomicrograph of biopsy from the maxillary sinus (23×, hematoxylin and eosin stain)* showing squamous cell carcinoma at the top. The rest of the tissue reveals extensive necrosis.

(G) *Photomicrograph of biopsy from the maxillary sinus of a different area than Figure 8F (24×)* reveals a sinus cavity lined by columnar epithelium with a focus of tumor (top left) and edematous subepithelial areas of chronic sinusitis at the bottom.

Case 9

SQUAMOUS CELL CARCINOMA OF THE EXTERNAL AUDITORY CANAL

Clinical presentation

A 48 year old male with no prior history of ear disease complained of severe left-sided headaches and left ear pain for four months. On examination, there was a white, exophytic, soft tissue mass in the external canal. The tympanic membrane could not be seen. Biopsy revealed a squamous cell carcinoma of the external canal.

Radiologic findings

CT of the temporal bones (bone window settings) with axial (Figure 9A) and coronal (Figure 9C) sections demonstrated a soft tissue mass in the left external auditory canal. There was partial erosion of the bony outline of the external canal as well as erosion of the anterior and superior mastoid and of the medial portion of the temporomandibular fossa.

The MRI axial (Figure 9B) and coronal (Figure 9D) projections demonstrated a soft tissue mass of intermediate SI and relatively high SI, respectively on T_1- and T_2-CW images.

Surgical and histopathological findings

A mastoidectomy procedure was performed (middle ear ossicles, and tympanic membrane were removed) and extended until a lateral bone resection was accomplished. The surgery encompassed the tumor mass, which seemed to extend from the external canal to the tympanic membrane, and posteriorly to the most anterior part of the mastoid air cells. Anteriorly, there was erosion with exposure of the temporomandibular joint (TMJ). The temporal bone defect was packed with fat [14] and the patient received postoperative radiation therapy.

The pathological examination of the specimen confirmed the presence of tumor in the external canal at the level of the tympanic membrane around the incus and malleus, and also in the TMJ. The rest of the anterior wall of the middle ear cavity was free of tumor. Histological examination of tumor tissue from the external canal showed squamous cell carcinoma of the surface mucosa with soft tissue extension associated with moderate fibrosis (Figure 9E). This tumor was focally cellular, keratinizing, and invasive.

Comments

Squamous cell carcinomas of the temporal bone usually arise at the junction of the middle ear and external canal. They are treated by surgical resection and postoperative radiation therapy [15].

CT is the method of choice for the evaluation of the temporal bone, due to its ability to generate high resolution images of bone that are necessary for evaluating the middle ear bone, ossicles, and bony facial canal. However, CT, unlike MRI, is unable to differentiate fluid in the ear from tumor. MRI's superior soft tissue contrast and multiplanar capability, along with its ability to delineate soft tissue components of tumor outside the temporal bone, makes it a valuable complementary tool for temporal bone imaging. Therefore, the evaluation of temporal bone tumors (carcinoma, sarcoma, glomus tumors, metastatic disease) should include CT, as a first step, followed by MR. MR has proved to be a helpful tool in the evaluation of the TMJ and adjacent anatomical areas [16].

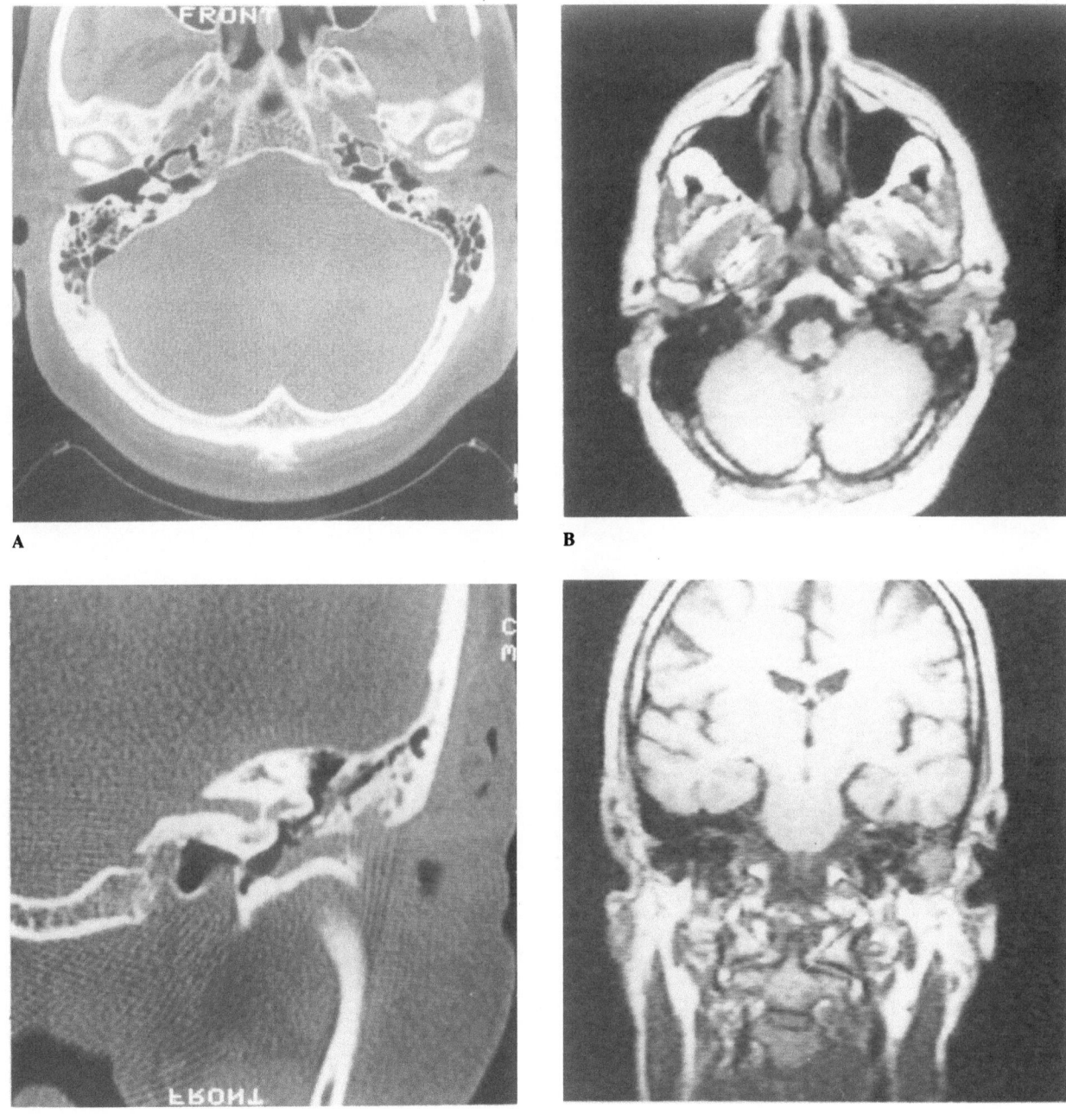

A

B

C

D

Figure 9. (A) *Axial contrast high resolution CT section at the level of the tympanic cavity* reveals a mass in the left external auditory canal and anterior middle ear cavity, with erosion of the anterior mastoid. There is mottled partial erosion of the bony external canal, along with some erosion of the anterior bony wall of the tympanic cavity.
(B) *Comparable axial MR projection (TR 400/TE 20 − NEX = 4; SLT = 0.5 cm)* reveals a mass of intermediate SI involving the external auditory canal and extending posteriorly to the mastoid air cells.

(C) *Coronal high resolution CT section through the tympanic cavity* shows a mass in the external auditory canal abutting and perforating the tympanic membrane with suggestion of extension into the middle ear cavity. There is erosion of the upper wall of the bony external canal and adjacent mastoid.
(D) *Comparable coronal MR projection (TR 400/TE 200 − NEX = 4; SLT = 0.5 cm).* The soft tissue mass of intermediate SI is localized in the bony external canal.

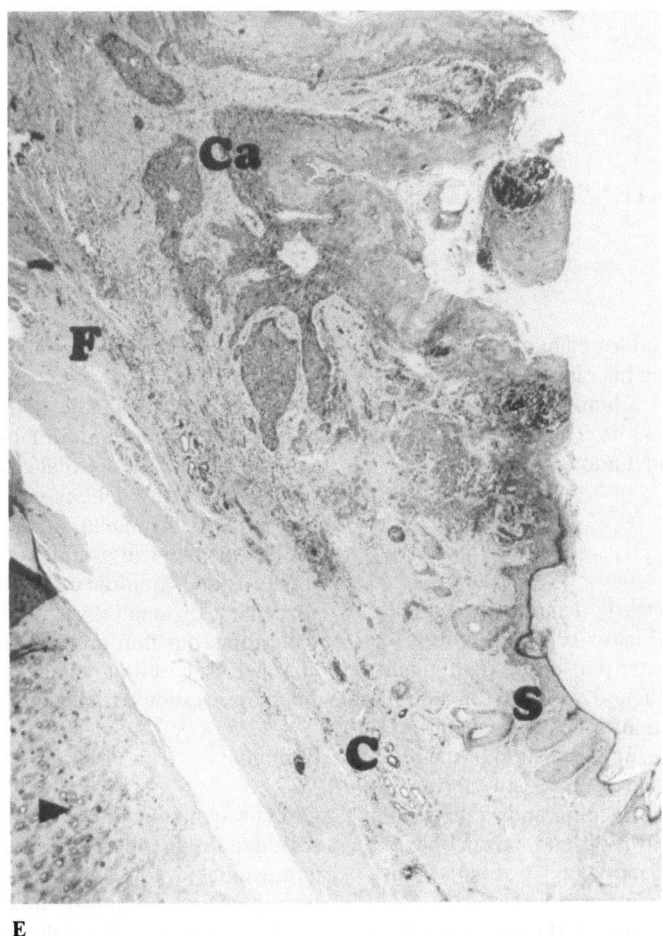

E

Figure 9. (E) *Photomicrograph of external ear canal* (31×, hematoxylin and eosin stain) shows squamous cell carcinoma (Ca) of the skin of the external canal (S). Note fibrosis (F), ceruminous glands (C) and cartilage of the ear canal (arrowhead).

Case 10

GLOMUS TYMPANICUM TUMOR
WITH EXTENSION INTO THE UPPER PART OF JUGULAR FOSSA

Clinical presentation

A 68 year old male complained for eight months of hearing loss and pulsatile tinnitus in his right ear. On examination, there was a reddish mass behind the tympanic membrane, with conductive hearing loss. The clinical diagnosis was a right glomus tympanicum tumor.

Radiologic findings

A high resolution CT study clearly demonstrated a mass in the right hypotympanum (Figure 10A). Moreover, the lower sections through the upper part of the right jugular fossa revealed irregular destruction with loss of the normal, well defined cortical margin, which was indicative of extension of the tumor into the upper portion of the jugular fossa (Figure 10A). Further sections inferiorly (not illustrated) revealed normal cortication and definition of the jugular fossa. The carotid canal and caroticojugular spine were well defined and appeared normal (Figure 10A).

Axial (Figure 10B) and coronal (Figure 10C) MR images demonstrated a small mass of intermediate SI on both T_1- and T_2-CW images. The mass was located in the right hypo- and mesotympanum, just cephalad to the entry of the internal jugular vein.

A selective arteriogram of the right external carotid artery (Figure 10D) confirmed the diagnosis of a hypervascular tumor consistent with glomus tympanicum tumor with extension into the upper jugular fossa. The tumor was fed chiefly by a posterior branch from the right ascending pharyngeal artery (Figure 10D). The tumor was embolized with polyvinyl alcohol particles.

Surgical and histopathological findings

A canal up mastoidectomy with posterior hypotympanotomy was performed and the tumor was removed. The tumor involved the hypotympanum, and extended anteriorly into the anterior hypotympanic air cells, and posteriorly into the retrofacial air cells of the mastoid. The jugular bulb was dehiscent and the tumor was in close proximity to the jugular bulb but did not invade it.

The histological examination of the small biopsy fragments from the middle ear and the jugular area showed replacement by small nests and clusters of cells associated with numerous thin walled blood vessels. The pattern was characteristic of a paraganglioma (glomus tumor). One of the biopsies showed extension of the tumor into bone.

Comments

Glomus tympanicum tumors can usually be completely resected. Frequently, glomus jugulare tumors are biopsied and irradiated, following mastoidectomy and fat obliteration, in order to minimize radionecrosis [14].

MR is superior for delineating soft tissue masses extending outside the temporal bone, including glomus jugulare tumors. Coronal MR images demonstrate the relationship of jugular fossa neoplasms to the jugular vein, which appears as a signal void. Neck extension is better appreciated on coronal and sagittal MR images.

However, CT gives better bone definition of temporal bone structures, and better assessment of bone destruction. Small glomus tympanic tumors are better defined with axial and coronal high resolution CT images. However, it should be noted that MRI, on T_1-CW images following the intravenous administration of Gd-DTPA [17] also delineates these small lesions. They enhance markedly and thereby contrast sharply with the surrounding signal void of bone and air.

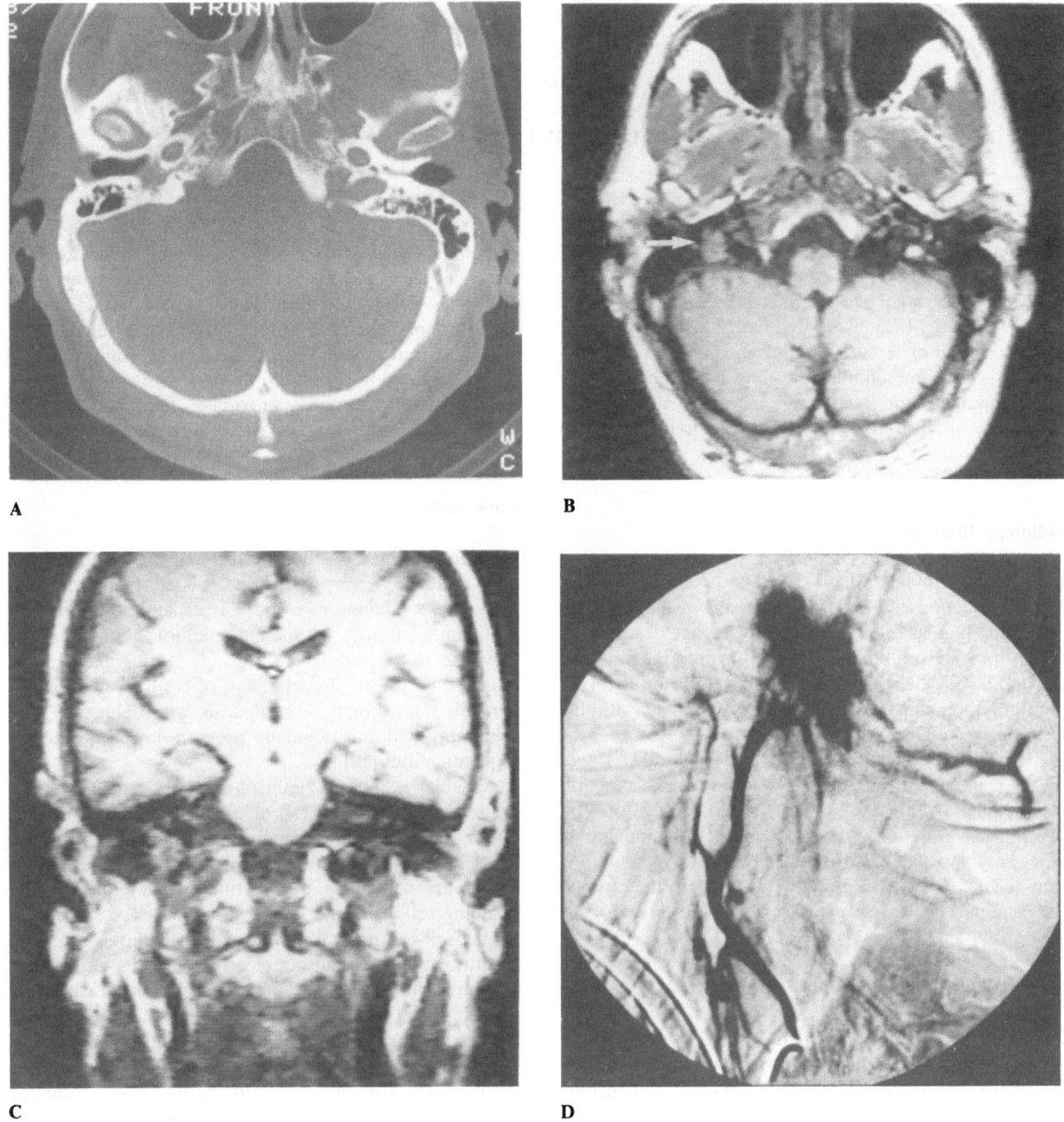

A

B

C

D

Figure 10. (A) *High resolution axial CT section through the hypotympanum* demonstrates a homogeneous mass within the right hypotympanum with invasion and destruction of the upper jugular fossa.
(B) *Comparable axial MR projection (TR 500/TE 21 − NEX = 4; SLT = 0.5 cm)* shows a 1-cm mass of intermediate SI in the middle ear (arrow).
(C) *Coronal MR projection at the level of the internal auditory*

canal (TR 400/TE 20 − NEX = 6; SLT = 0.4 cm). The mass extends from the middle ear cavity inferiorly into the jugular foramen. The exact inferior limit on this relatively low resolution study cannot be determined.
(D) Pre-embolization selective angiogram of the right ascending pharyngeal artery. Selective injection of the external carotid artery reveals dilatation of the ascending pharyngeal artery with a dense tumor blush of the glomus tympanicum tumor.

49

Case 11

GLOMUS JUGULARE TUMOR

Clinical presentation

A 27 year old woman over the past 2–3 years had noticed ringing in her right ear, associated with a throbbing sensation, which had increased in both frequency and intensity over the last several months. A lesion was seen behind the right tympanic membrane. It was biopsied via tympanotomy and, on histological examination, found to be a glomus tumor.

Radiologic findings

A CT study with axial (Figure 11A) and coronal (Figures 11C & D) sections showed a large, enhancing mass arising in the right jugular fossa, causing diffuse bone destruction within the temporal bone and extending into the mastoid and middle ear cavity, as well as into the posterior fossa. In addition, the mass extended to the upper neck with the lower border not clearly defined on CT.

MRI with axial (Figure 11B), coronal (Figure 11E), and sagittal (Figure 11F) projections demonstrated a mass of intermediate SI on T_1-CW images and of high SI on T_2-CW images, with linear areas of signal void, indicating either vascularity or calcification. The mass expanded the right jugular fossa and invaded the right infratemporal fossa and middle ear with extension to the posterior fossa.

Treatment and histological considerations

The radiologic studies showed that the lesion was large (almost 3 cm in greatest dimension) and extended over approximately 3 cm in the superoinferior dimension. Moreover, because of the patient's age, the strategic location of the lesion, and its relatively benign nature, radiotherapy was preferred over surgery. She was given 44.8 Gy, in eighteen fractions, over twenty-eight days.

Glomus jugulare and glomus tympanicum tumors belong to the subgroup of jugulotympanic paragangliomas. Paraganglion cells can be located in the adventitia of the anterior part of the dome of the jugular bulb (paraganglion or glomus jugulare) or in the middle ear (paraganglion or glomus tympanicum) [18]. These tumors are composed of chief cells in nests or balls, surrounded by numerous thin walled vascular channels. Occasionally, these vascular channels are thrombosed, producing areas of fibrosis within the tumor. These chief cells can vary in configuration and size, but usually have a regular and orderly arrangement, often herniating into vascular spaces, simulating glomeruli. The diagnosis of this tumor is supported by immunoperoxidase stains and electron microscopic studies showing dense core granules.

Comments

CT demonstrates the bony erosion in the jugular fossa and remaining temporal bone better than MRI. A markedly enhancing mass on CT, expanding the jugular foramen is almost pathognomonic for glomus tumor. However, in this case, there was only slight enhancement, most likely due to slow infusion of contrast material. A dynamic scan should be carried out with bolus injection, preferably with an automatic pressure injector, and fast sequential films [19].

Vascular lesions in the head and neck have no blood-brain barrier, and infusion of contrast material from the tumor into the adjacent tissue does not take place. Increased contrast accumulation can only be demonstrated within the capillaries of the tumor. Therefore, instant scanning following the injection is necessary to demonstrate peak contrast values within the capillaries.

In this case, CT did not clearly depict the inferior extension of the tumor. MRI, due to its multiplanar capability and improved soft tissue contrast, detected the extent of the lesion into the upper neck and its intracranial extension. MRI detected the soft tissue component of this lesion in great detail, especially on the T_2-CW images. Moreover, the location in the jugular fossa and the presence of signal voids, representing vascular channels on MR images, was very suggestive of a glomus tumor [20]. Additionally, the use of fast imaging techniques and Gd-DTPA make it possible to detect even smal paragangliomas in the temporal bone [17].

In summary, when there is clinical suspicion of jugular fossa pathology, MRI with Gd-DTPA should be the first study to be performed. However, if the study is inconclusive, especially in regard to bone destruction or a small mass in the hypo/mesotympanum, high resolution CT

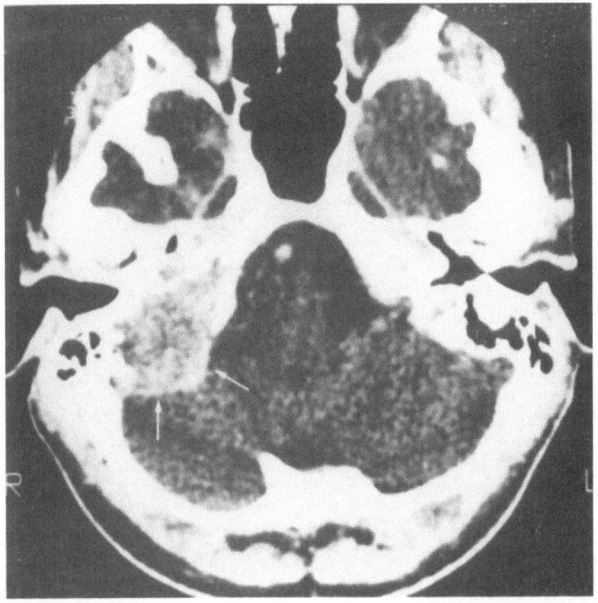

A

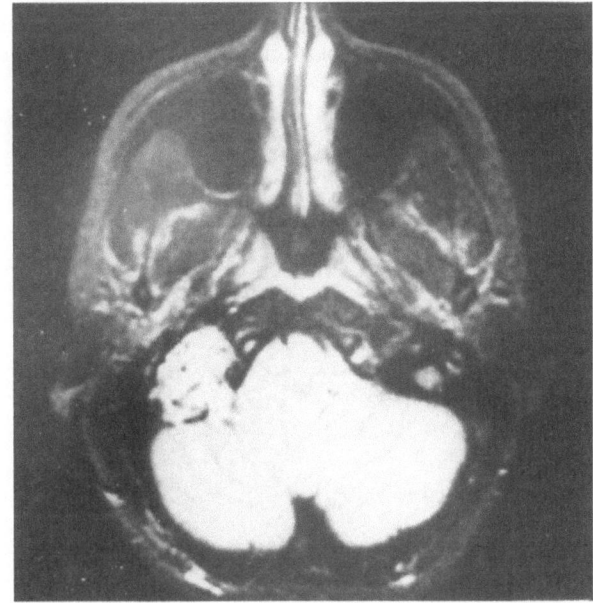

B

Figure 11. (A) *Axial contrast CT section through the mid portion of the temporal bone* reveals a homogeneous, slightly enhancing mass in the region of the right jugular fossa with extension into the right posterior fossa and extensive bone destruction about the jugular fossa. Tumor impresses on the right cerebellar hemisphere without evidence of invasion (arrow).

(B) *Axial MR image at a similar level (TR 2220/TE 80 − NEX = 1; SLT = 0.5 cm)* shows a heterogeneous mass of predominantly high SI with internal, linear low SI areas, centered within the right jugular fossa, with invasion of the posterior fossa.

C. Temporal bone/base of skull

should be added. This is particularly relevant in cases where on otoscopy a pinkish mass is seen in the middle ear cavity.

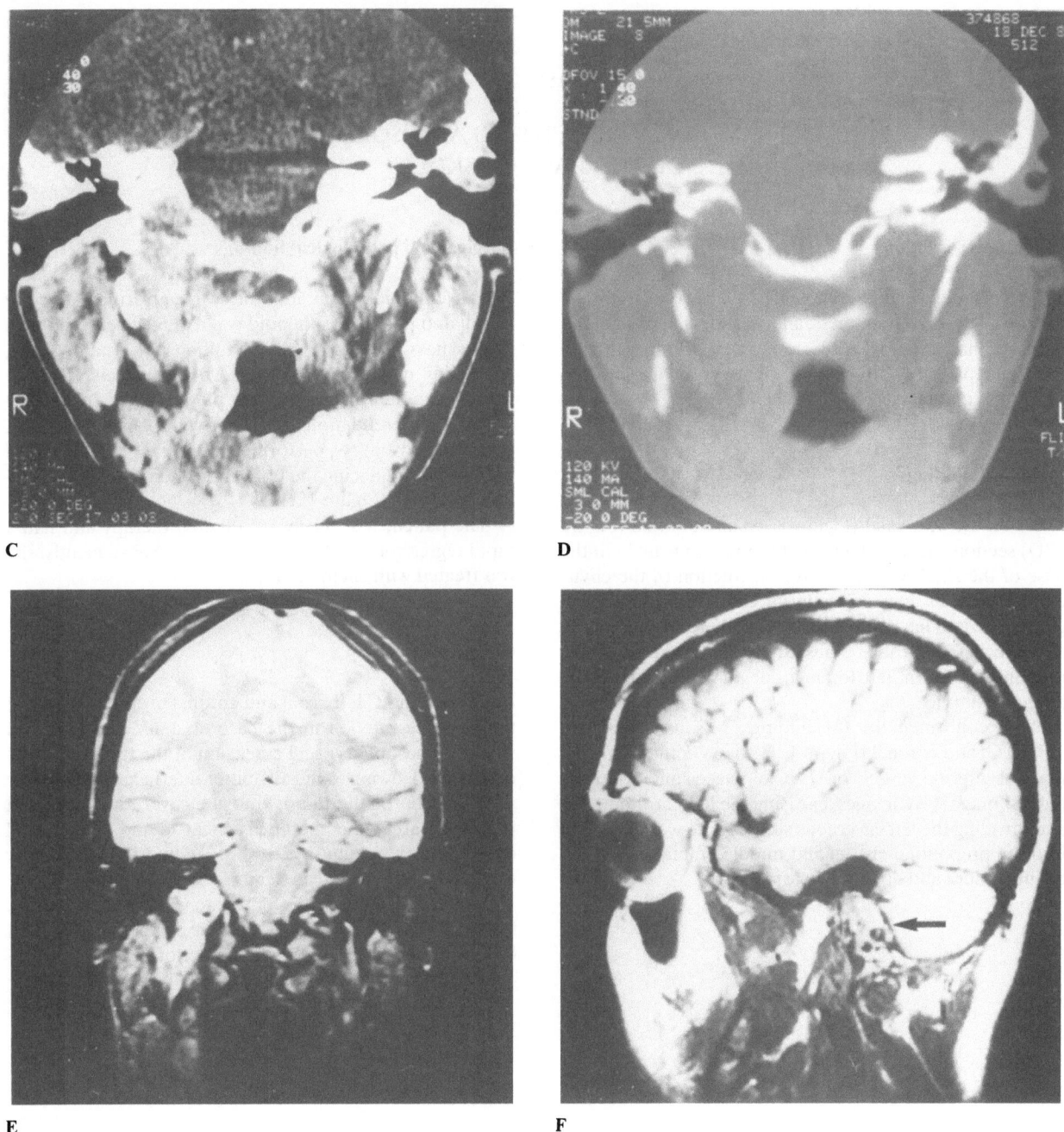

C

D

E

F

Figure 11.(C & D) *Coronal contrast CT section including bone window setting at the level of the internal auditory canal* reveals a slightly enhancing, ill-defined mass within the jugular fossa with extension into the upper neck. There is erosion of the jugular fossa, including the undersurface of the right petrous bone. There is minimal projection of the mass into the hypotympanum. **(E)** *Coronal MR image at the level of the internal auditory canal (TR 2300/TE 80 − NEX = 1; SLT = 0.5 cm).* There is a large

mass of high SI with linear low SI areas expanding the right jugular foramen and extending inferiorly into the upper neck.
(F) *Right parasagittal MR image (TR 570/TE 20 − NEX = 1; SLT = 0.5 cm)* reveals a mass of intermediate SI containing areas of low SI expanding right jugular fossa, bulging into posterior aspect of the mastoid with resulting impression on the anterior aspect of the cerebellar hemisphere. There is no evidence of invasion of dura or cerebellar hemisphere (arrow).

53

Case 12

MULTIPLE MYELOMA PRESENTING AS A SOLITARY LESION OF THE BASE OF SKULL

Clinical presentation

A 75 year old woman complained for several weeks of diplopia, left facial numbness, and weakness. On examination, she had bilateral VIth nerve palsy along with left IVth and partial VIIth palsies. Conductive hearing loss was found on the left side.

Radiologic findings

A CT study, with axial (Figure 12A) and coronal (Figure 12D) sections, revealed a large, homogeneous mass in the base of the skull, with extensive destruction of the clivus and left petrous apex, left anterior clinoid process, pterygoid bone, and left occipital condyle. There was extension into the left cavernous sinus, sella, left sphenoid sinus, prepontine cistern, left foramen magnum, and the upper left nasopharynx.

MRI confirmed the CT findings. MR axial (Figures 12B & C) and coronal (Figure 12E) views demonstrated a mass of intermediate SI on T_1-CW images and relatively high SI on T_2-CW images, encasing the left carotid artery and invading the left cavernous sinus. There was extension into the prepontine cistern and middle cranial fossa with an intact dura and no brain invasion.

Surgical and pathological findings

A transethmoid sphenoidotomy was performed. The left lateral and posterior sphenoid walls were absent. Biopsies of the mass showed a cellular tumor with scant stroma, containing numerous thin-walled blood vessels. The cellular component consisted of plasma cells in varying stages of differentiation consistent with plasmacytoma. A bone marrow biopsy, performed a few days later, revealed plasma cells replacing the bone marrow, indicative of multiple myeloma (Figure 12F).

The patient first received radiation therapy and had a rapid regression of all of her symptoms. Subsequently, she was treated with chemotherapy.

Comments

Both MRI and CT, in axial and coronal projections, reveal the bone destruction in the base of skull. The sphenoid sinus and nasopharyngeal extension of the tumor are well demarcated, owing to the air-tumor interface.

Extension of the tumor into the cavernous sinus and parasellar area, and the encasement of the left internal carotid artery by tumor are well seen by MRI, but not by CT. MRI, but not CT, can demonstrate the intact dura.

In this case, MRI was superior to CT in tumor staging. CT now plays a secondary role in evaluating the skull base. However, CT should still be performed in questionable cases of subtle erosion of the skull base [21].

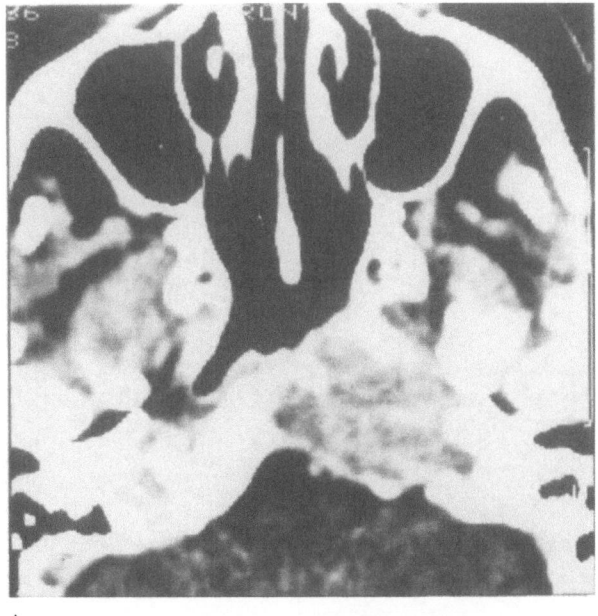

A

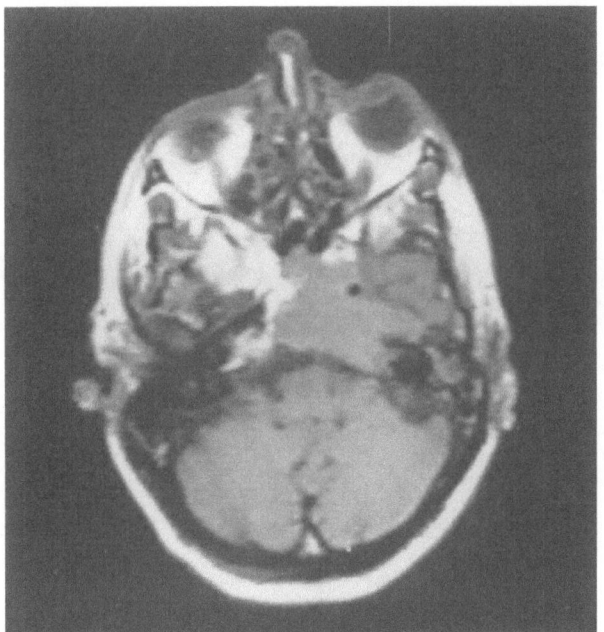

B

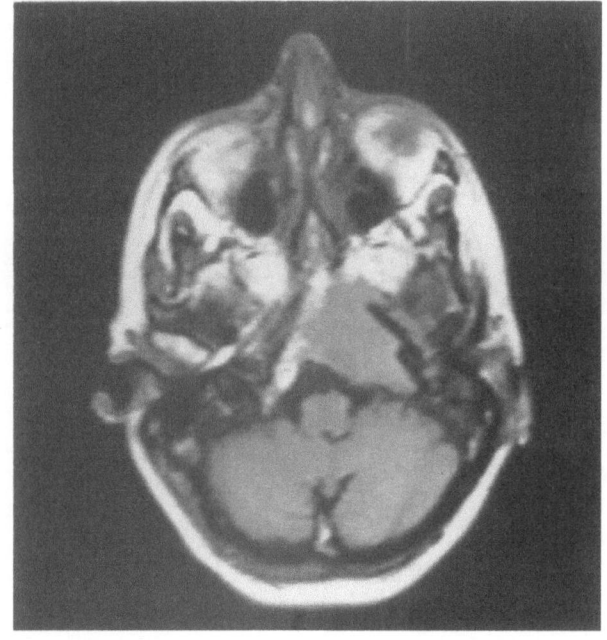

C

Figure 12. (A) *Axial contrast CT section through the nasopharynx* reveals a mass in the base of skull with erosion of the left clivus and apex of the left petrous pyramid. The mass extends into the prepontine cistern and left nasopharynx.
(B & C) *Axial MR comparable projections (TR 500/TE 21 − NEX = 6; SLT = 0.5 cm).* A mass of intermediate SI invades the clivus and the left petrous apex. The tumor invades the posterior aspect of the left sphenoid sinus (Figure 12B) and encases, but does not narrow, the petrous portion of the left carotid artery. The marrow of the right petrous apex exhibits a normally high SI. The mass enters the left prepontine cistern and left middle cranial fossa (Figure 12C) without invasion of dura, verified on T_2-CW images (not shown).

55

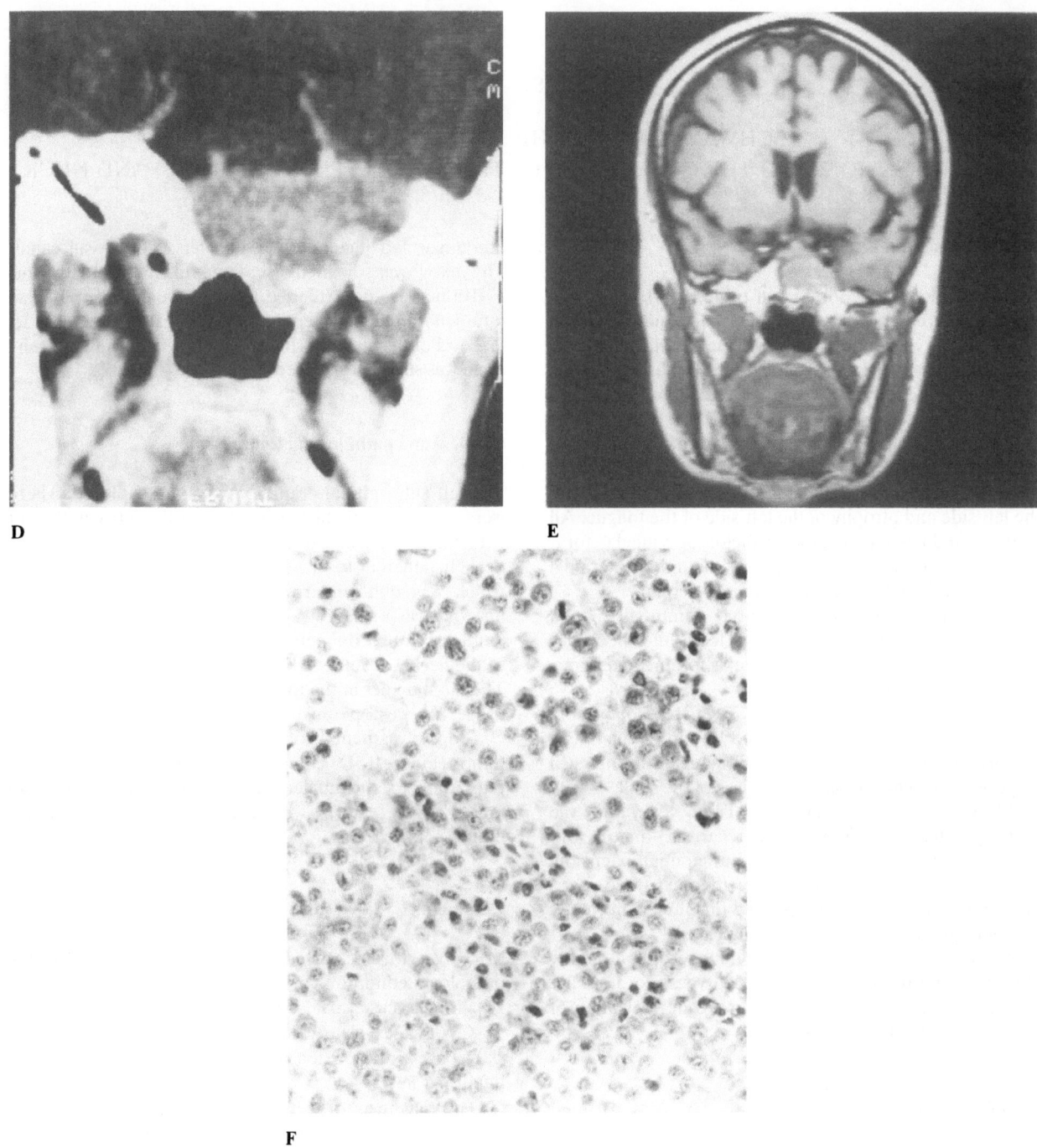

D

E

F

Figure 12.(D) *Coronal contrast CT section through the naso-pharynx* demonstrates the mass in the base of skull with erosion of the clivus and left petrous apex, with extension into the upper left portion of the nasopharynx.
(E) *Comparable coronal MR projection (TR 500/TE 21 − NEX = 6; SLT = 0.5 cm).* A mass of intermediate SI invades the left cavernous sinus abutting the carotid artery. The pituitary stalk and gland are compressed inferiorly. The mass is in close prox-imity to the left temporal lobe, but separated from it by an intact dark line representing the dura.
(F) *Photomicrograph from a bone marrow biopsy (400 ×, Giem-sa)* shows replacement of bone marrow by immature plasma cells with eccentrically placed nuclei.

C. Temporal bone/base of skull

Case 13

SCHWANNOMA OF THE JUGULAR FORAMEN
WITH EXTENSION INTO THE CEREBELLOPONTINE ANGLE, PETROUS BONE, AND NECK

Clinical presentation

A 33 year old man reported that twelve years previously he noted a gradual weakening of his voice and was found to have a left vocal cord paralysis. Since an initial investigation did not reveal a cause for this 10th nerve palsy, he underwent a Teflon injection of the vocal cord, which improved his voice.

Five years later, he developed weakness of his left shoulder and, on examination, aside from vocal cord paralysis, there was a slight diminution of the gag reflex on the left side and atrophy of the left side of the tongue. All of these findings aroused the suspicion of a jugular foramen syndrome (lesion of the IXth, Xth, and XIth cranial nerves), combined with XIIth nerve involvement.

A CT study demonstrated a large, dumb-bell shaped tumor extending from the posterior fossa into the upper neck. There was erosion of the jugular foramen and apex of the petrous bone.

Subsequently, the patient had a two-stage operation, consisting of a craniotomy, followed by extracranial neck exploration. The tumor was excised and the histological diagnosis was schwannoma of the base of the skull.

CT scans were done annually. Three years after the first operation, a CT revealed recurrent tumor with erosion of the petrous bone, and intracranial extension. The tumor enlarged gradually over the next three years. Over this time period, the patient functioned normally without significant worsening of symptoms.

The examination upon admission for re-operation disclosed slight VIth nerve weakness, left vocal cord paralysis, wasting of the left trapezius muscle, and deviation of the tongue to the left.

Radiologic findings

MRI was performed and T_1- and T_2-CW images were obtained in both the axial (Figure 13A) and coronal (Figures 13B & C) projections. MRI demonstrated a mass of intermediate SI on T_1-CW images and of high SI on T_2-CW images (Figures 13A, B & C within the left cerebellopon-

tine angle, left jugular fossa, and left hypoglossal canal. The mass was distinctly separate from the VIIth and VIIIth nerves and extended through the enlarged jugular foramen into the adjacent soft tissues of the upper neck to the level of the alveolar ridge of the maxilla. The IVth ventricle was slightly displaced towards the right.

Surgical and pathological findings

The left suboccipital craniotomy was re-explored. There were adhesions of thickened dura to the left cerebellum with loculations of proteinaceous fluid. The tumor was densely adherent to the dura around the jugular foramen, which was quite enlarged. The inferior portion of the mastoid was drilled away and that portion of tumor extending through the petrous bone and into the soft tissue of the neck was removed under the operating microscope. The large defect in the inferior mastoid was filled with fat tissue. The postoperative course was uneventful.

Biopsy fragments from the jugular foramen showed a tumor (Figure 13D) composed of spindle cells with focal palisading of the nuclei and occasional loose, myxoid areas. These features were characteristics of a schwannoma [22].

Comments

MRI has already proved to be a superior modality for pathologic conditions of the cerebellopontine angle [23–24]. In this case, axial and coronal images (particularly T_2-CW images) clearly demonstrated the lesion within the skull base and its extension into the posterior fossa and left upper neck.

The diagnosis of schwannoma was suggested by the absence of increased vascularity (serpiginous signal void areas), which would have favored a glomus tumor (the only other likely entity in the differential diagnosis). The presence of an intact jugular vein was also an argument against the diagnosis of glomus tumor.

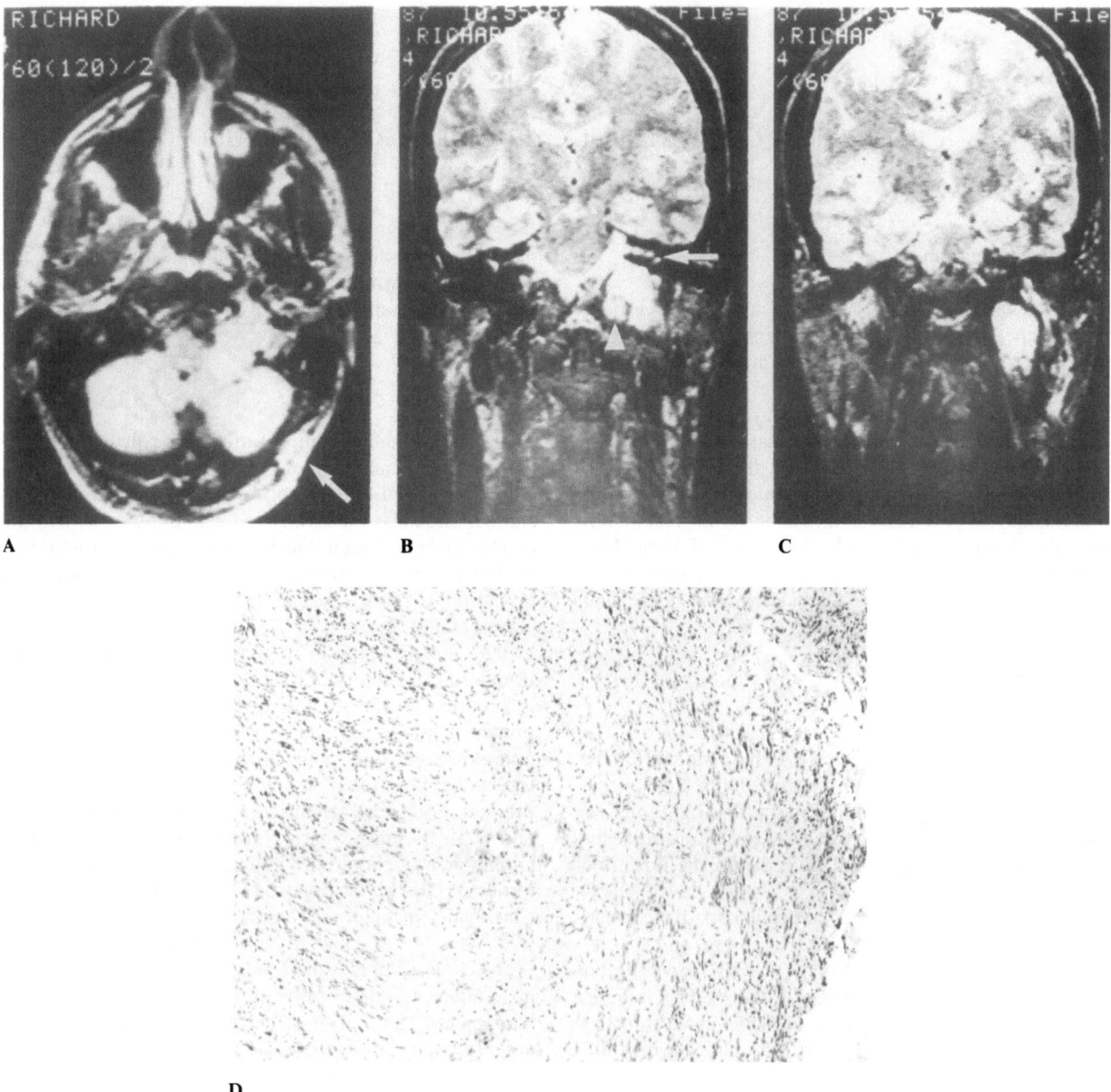

Figure 13.(A) *Axial MR projection at the level of the jugular foramen (TR 2000/TE 60 – NEX = 2; SLT = 0.4 cm).* A mass of high SI is located in the left jugular foramen, extending into the petrous apex and jugular fossa, with encroachment upon the left cerebellar hemisphere posteriorly. The mass displaces the left carotid artery anteriorly, abuts the longus colli muscle medially and extends to the mastoid air cells laterally. There is an area of high SI (arrow) on this mildly T_2-CW image (intermediate SI on T_1-CW image) in the left occipital subcutaneous tissue, compatible with proteinaceous fluid or soft tissue with high water content. These changes correspond to the location of the previous craniotomy.

(B & C) *Coronal MR projections at the level of the internal auditory canal (TR 2000/TE 120 – NEX = 2; SLT = 0.4 cm).* The mass of high SI is demonstrated in the left jugular fossa, invading or eroding the occipital condyle (arrowhead). The internal auditory canal (arrow) is normal (Figure 13B). The tumor extends inferiorly into the upper neck, displacing the internal jugular vein laterally (Figure 13C).

(D) *Photomicrograph of biopsy fragment from jugular foramen (100×, hematoxylin and eosin stain)* showing the schwannoma with a myxoid stroma.

59

Case 14

RECURRENT CHOLESTEROL CYST OF THE BASE OF SKULL

Clinical presentation

A 54 year old man had a fourteen year history of a right petrous apex cyst, for which he underwent multiple surgical procedures. Initially, a middle cranial fossa drainage was performed, followed fifteen months later by a left ethmoid trans-sphenoid approach to the right petrous apex. The cyst was marsupialized with a nasal septal mucosal flap. In order to secure persistent drainage, a silastic drainage tube had to be inserted three times, twice at intervals of two years, and a third time, seven years later, since the drainage track had healed over with bone. Sixteen months after the last operation, the patient once again presented with severe headaches and a right facial nerve palsy.

Radiologic findings

The CT study with axial (Figure 14A) and coronal (Figure 14C) sections demonstrated a sharply defined, isodense, ring enhancing, extra-axial lesion in the right middle cranial fossa with bone erosion. The mass was adjacent to the right petrous apex and bulged into the posterior fossa.

An MRI, performed with axial (Figure 14B), coronal (Figure 14D), and sagittal projections, showed a 3 cm, extra-axial mass with a low SI rim on T_2-CW images and a uniform high SI center on both T_1- and T_2-CW images. The cyst arose in the base of skull and bulged into the right middle cranial fossa, and via the incisura into the prepontine cistern.

Surgical and pathological considerations

The clinical picture, as well as the MR and CT findings, on sequential follow-up examinations, were suggestive of reaccumulation of fluid with consequent enlargement of the cyst, prompting revision surgery. Using the operating microscope, the right sphenoid cavity was visualized and the posterior sphenoid drilled through thick bone to the level of the cyst that was located in the right middle cranial fossa adjacent to the petrous apex. The cyst was loculated and a large volume of thick, brown-gold liquid

material was evacuated. The pathological analysis of the gelatinous, brown material showed proteinaceous debris, red blood cells, and cholesterol clefts.

Comments

The CT examination demonstrated a sharply defined, isodense, nonenhancing lesion. The appearance was consistent with a cyst, but a neurogenic tumor could not be excluded. The mass was associated with bony erosion in the petrous apex and, on a statistical basis, an epidermoid or a cholesterol cyst was the most likely possibility. Intra-axial brain tumors rarely cause destruction of the skull table or base of skull.

The bony erosion in the base of skull is better illustrated on CT with a bone window setting. However, MRI is superior to CT for visualizing the intracranial component of the lesion and its relationship to the adjacent temporal lobe and pons. MRI, also characterizes this lesion as a fluid filled cyst, containing blood degradation products and its MR signal characteristics (high SI on T_1- and T_2-CW images) are considered as almost pathognomonic of a cholesterol granuloma [25] or of a cholesterol cyst [26–27], as opposed to an epidermoid cyst [28]. Classically, the epidermoid cyst evokes intermediate SI on T_1-CW images and high SI on T_2-CW images. The high SI of the cholesterol cyst on T_1-CW images is a reflection of its content (golden-brownish, gelatinous material containing cholesterol crystals, chronic hemorrhage products and proteinaceous debris).

The etiology of petrous apex cystic lesions is a subject of some controversy [26–27, 29]. Congenital or primary epidermoid cyst refers to a squamous epithelium-lined cyst filled with keratin debris; whereas a cholesterol granuloma or giant cholesterol cyst has no epithelial lining, should not contain any squamous cell debris, and has only a fibrous wall. This differentiation has surgical importances: (1) the goal in the treatment of a cholesterol cyst of the temporal bone is permanent drainage and not total surgical removal, since there is no distinct epithelial lining; and (2) an epidermoid cyst requires complete removal of the epithelial lining after evacuation of the keratin debris to forestall continuous desquamation of epithelial cells.

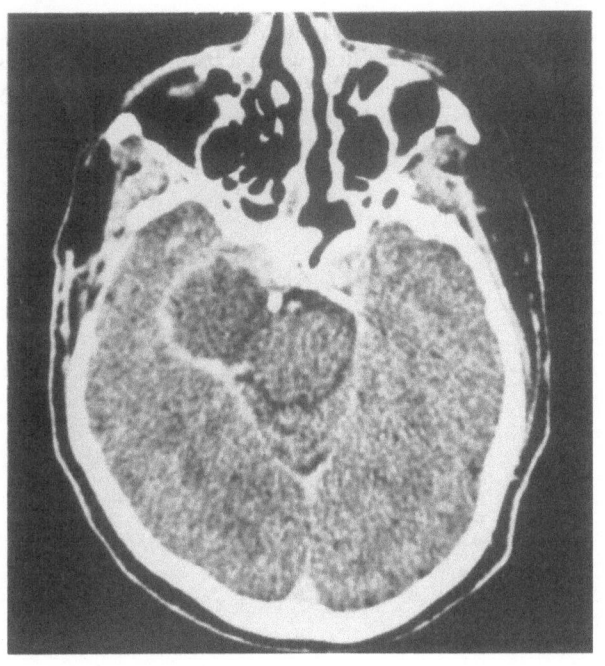

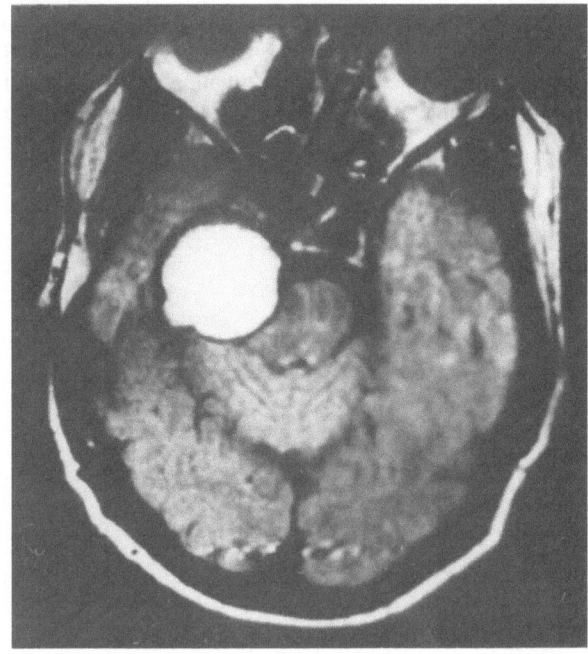

A   B

Figure 14. (A) *Axial contrast CT section through the level slightly above the base of skull* shows a large, well demarcated, ring-enhancing lesion in the right middle cranial fossa bulging via the incisura into the prepontine cistern. The lesion is isodense with brain. The enhancing rim is sharply marginated and represents enhancing dura. There is a lateral craniotomy defect at the level of the right greater wing of the sphenoid bone.

(B) *Axial MR projection at a comparable level (TR 2000/TE 35 − NEX = 1; SLT = 0.5 cm).* On this proton density-CW image, there is a 3 cm, high SI, extra-axial mass within the middle cranial fossa and prepontine cistern, without adjacent edema. There is slight indentation of the pons on the right. The mass has a thin peripheral ring of low SI corresponding to dura and a central region of uniform high SI.

61

C. Temporal bone/base of skull

In conclusion, MRI and CT were complementary in the diagnosis and demarcation of this cystic lesion. MR signal characteristics allow differentiation of a solid tumor from a cyst and, in most cases, can separate an epidermoid from a cholesterol cyst. MR is superior to CT and should be performed first, when a base of skull lesion is suspected. This should be followed by CT, if there is any question of bone involvement.

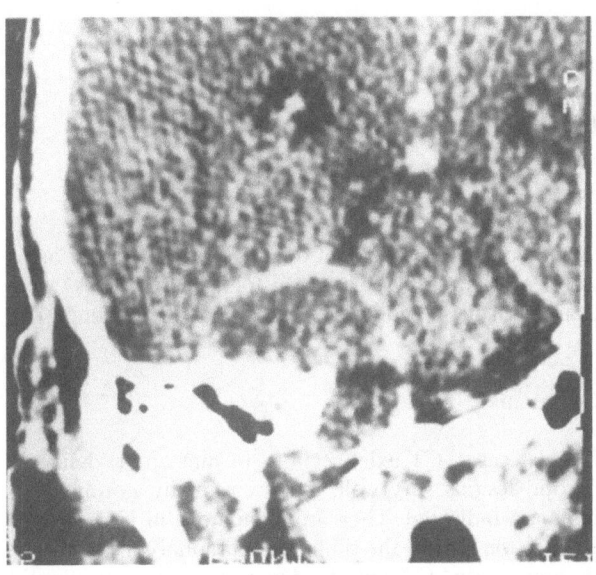

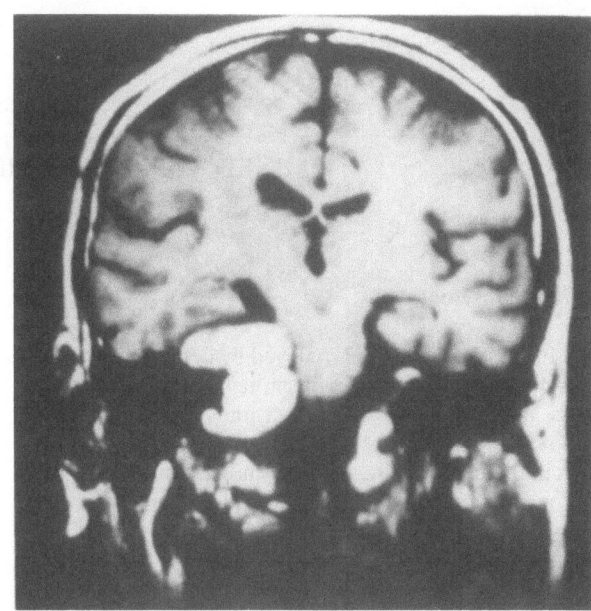

C

D

Figure 14. (C) *Coronal contrast CT section through the petrous pyramid* demonstrates the same ring-enhancing mass adjacent to the apex of the right petrous pyramid, bulging through the incisura into the posterior fossa, with encroachment on the pontine cistern.

(D) *Coronal MR projection at a comparable level* (*TR 600/TE 20 − NEX = 2; SLT = 0.5 cm*) shows an extra-axial mass eroding the right petrous apex, with a uniform high SI. The lesion encroaches upon the pons on the right.

63

Case 15

MIXED TUMOR OF THE LEFT PAROTID GLAND

Clinical presentation

A 34 year old woman was referred by her dentist, because of a mass in her left upper neck, below the earlobe. This mass had doubled in size over a four year period. There was no history of facial weakness or pain, but some soreness in the region of the mass was noted three weeks prior to consultation. On clinical examination there was a 2 cm, mobile, solid mass in the inferior portion of the left parotid gland.

Radiologic findings

A CT study, with axial (Figure 15A) sections was performed without contrast material, due to the patient's history of sensitivity to iodine. The examination showed an isodense lesion in the superficial portion of the left parotid gland.

MRI, with axial (Figures 15B, C & D) and coronal (Figure 15E) projections clearly outlined a mass within the superficial portion of the left parotid gland with intermediate SI on T_1-CW images and high SI on T_2-CW images. The sharp borders of the mass suggested a benign lesion.

Surgical and pathological findings

The patient underwent a left superficial parotidectomy. A smooth, encapsulated, 2 cm, bluish mass was found in the lower third of the parotid gland, which was dissected from the mandibular branch of the facial nerve.

A section through the surgical specimen disclosed a tumor mass sharply separated from the normal parotid tissue (Figure 15F) with scant focal peripheral fibrosis ('pseudocapsule'). The tumor was composed predominantly of a myxoid stroma with scattered areas of myoepi-

thelial cells and occasional ducts. Focal chondroid areas were also present. These histological findings were characteristic of pleomorphic adenoma (mixed tumor).

Comments

In most cases, CT axial sections (4 mm apart) delineate parotid lesions very well, but occasionally, coronal sections are indicated. They are mandatory in large lesions close to the base of the skull or in parapharyngeal tumors. In some cases, CT fails to demonstrate an intraparotid lesion, especially in patients with dense parotid glands. In these cases, there is insufficient contrast between the normally, low density parotid gland and the tumor.

MRI, with axial and coronal projections, optimally outlines parotid lesions and is probably the imaging method of choice for salivary gland tumors [30–31]. In our opinion, the MR strategy of parotid imaging should include coronal T_1-CW images (to define the superior and inferior borders of the lesion), in addition to the axial T_1- and T_2-CW images. In order to save time, T_2-CW images of localized regions can be obtained (Figure 15D) with gradient echo technique [32–33].

MRI was clearly superior to CT in this case. It was able to suggest the close relationship of the tumor to the mandibular branch of the facial nerve, since the tumor abutted the vessels (nerve is lateral to vessels). Using high resolution techniques, direct imaging of the intraparotid portion of the facial nerve is possible [34].

In this case, the MR signal intensity of the tumor was high on T_2-CW images, which was consistent with the presence of a predominant myxoid stroma in the tumor. The myxoid stroma is rich in hyaluronic acid produced by myoepithelial cells and is biochemically similar to a proteinaceous solution. The high water content of chondroid tissue also contributes to the high SI observed on T_2-CW images in pleomorphic adenomas [35].

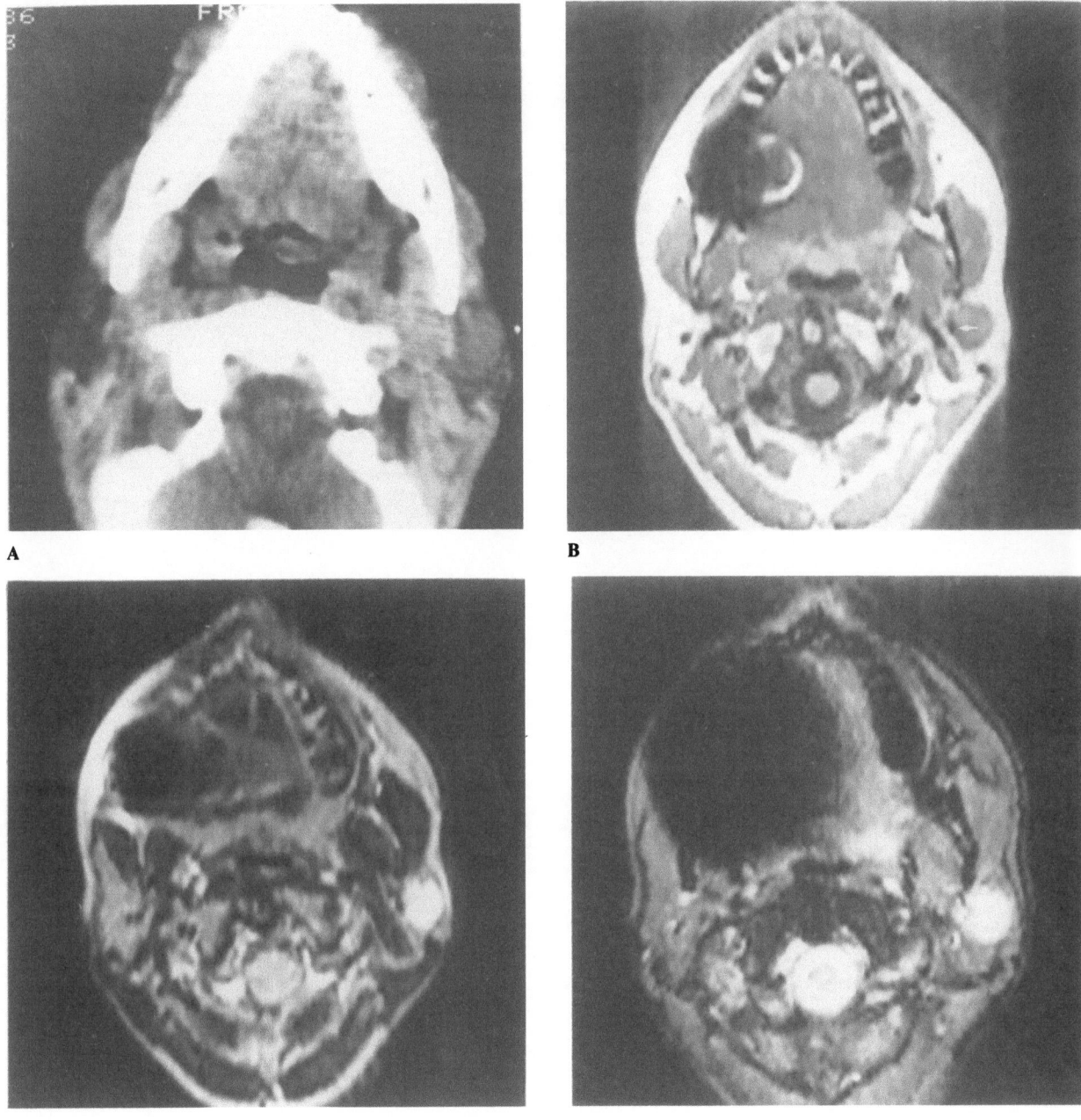

A

B

C

D

Figure 15. (A) *Axial CT section (without contrast) through the mid third of the parotid glands* shows an oval-shaped lesion (iso-dense with muscle) in the superficial portion of the left parotid gland, measuring 1.5 to 2 cm in greatest diameter.
(B) *Axial MR projection* (T_1-CW image) at comparable level *TR* 400/*TE* 21 − NEX = 6; SLT = 0.5 cm) demonstrates a well circumscribed mass of intermediate SI within the superficial lobe of the left parotid gland, adjacent to the lateral aspect of the retromandibular vein (RMV) (arrow).
(C & D) *Identical axial MR projections* (T_2-CW images) [(15C) spin echo, *TR* 2000/*TE* 96 − NEX = 4. SLT = 0.5 cm; (15D) gradient echo − low pulse flip angle (θ = 30°), *TR* 100/*TE* 30 −

NEX = 4; SLT = 0.7 cm] demonstrates the same mass within the superficial lobe of the left parotid gland with high SI. A dental amalgam causes a magnetic susceptibility-induced signal loss artifact in the region of the right alveolar ridge [5]. The signal loss is more pronounced with gradient echo (GRE) imaging (Figure 15D), which is more sensitive to magnetic susceptibility differences. GRE imaging of the parotid lesion has generated a T_2-CW image with a high SI in less than one minute, compared to the 17 minutes necessary to obtain a spin echo long *TR*/long *TE* image. However, only one slice was obtained in the GRE sequence, whereas 11 slices were obtained in the spin echo sequence.
(Figures 15B, C & D are reproduced with permission from [32].)

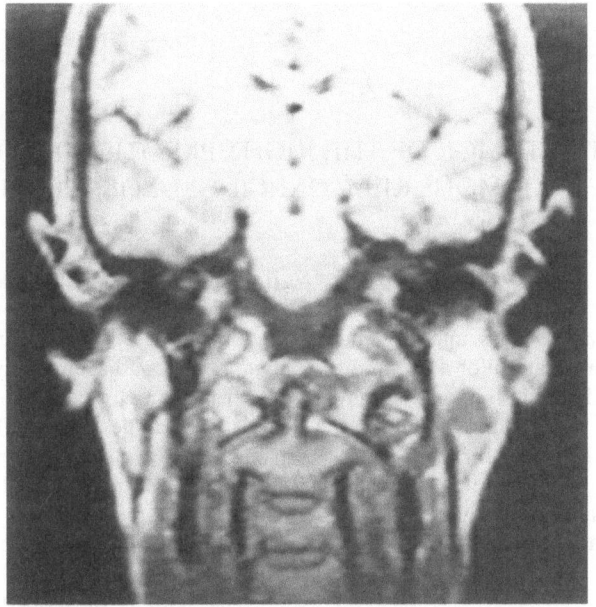

E

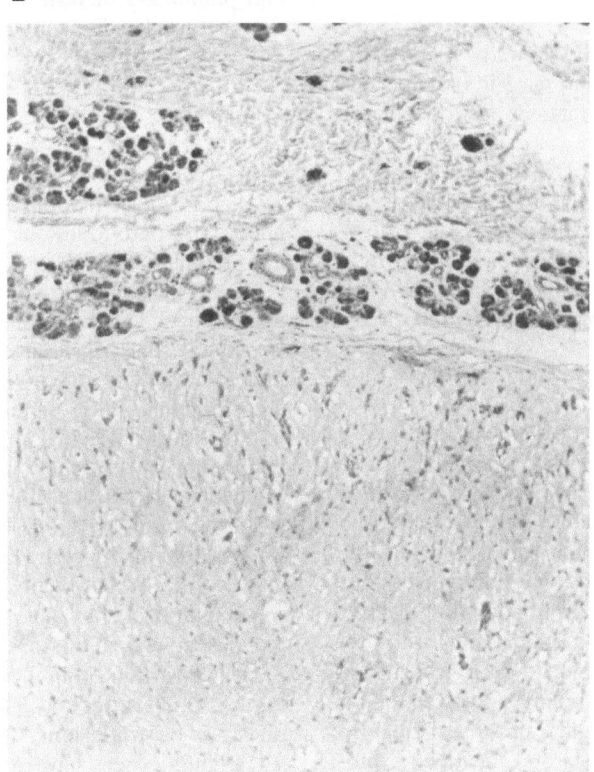

F

Figure 15. (E) *Coronal MR projection (TR 400/TE 20 − NEX = 6; SLT = 0.5 cm).* The mass of low SI contrasts with the higher SI of the parotid tissue, lateral to the RMV, and is located in the superficial portion of the parotid gland (facial nerve is lateral to RMV and represents the dividing line between the deep and superficial part of the parotid gland).

(F) *Photomicrograph of mixed tumor of the parotid gland (70 ×, hematoxylin and eosin stain)* shows normal parotid tissue at the top, replaced by tumor with abundant myxoid stroma and occasional myoepithelial cells.

Case 16

WARTHIN'S TUMOR OF THE RIGHT PAROTID GLAND AND METASTATIC SQUAMOUS CELL CARCINOMA OF THE RIGHT NECK

Clinical presentation

A 55 year old man had a right parotid mass, unchanged in size for two years. He sought consultation for a two and a half week history of swelling and pain in the right ear and preauricular area. Examination revealed a 6 × 8 cm, mobile, nontender mass involving the lower third and superficial lobe of the parotid gland and extending deep into the retromandibular area. No facial nerve weakness was noted. The ENT examination was otherwise normal.

Radiologic findings

A CT sialogram (Figures 16A & D) showed a lesion in the right parotid gland, and an irregular mass in the mid right neck that was consistent with matted, necrotic lymph nodes.

An MRI, with axial (Figures 16B, C, & E) and coronal projections demonstrated a well circumscribed lesion within the right parotid gland with high SI on T_2-CW images, along with a large, soft tissue mass in the right neck displacing the neurovascular bundle medially. This tumor had heterogeneous, intermediate to high SI on T_2-CW images.

Surgical and histological findings

A needle biopsy of the right neck mass was performed and yielded squamous cell carcinoma with giant cells and rare foci of keratinization (Figure 16F). A biopsy of the parotid gland revealed acute and chronic inflammation.

The patient was initially treated with radiation therapy, and then underwent a right total parotidectomy with preservation of the facial nerve combined with a right radical neck dissection (RND). The parotid mass involved the lower third of the superficial lobe with extension to the deep lobe. No tumor was found in the carotid sheath on exploration of the neck.

The histopathologic examination of the surgical specimens showed an adenolymphoma (Warthin's tumor) in the parotid gland that was altered by fibrosis secondary to radiation. The tumor was cystic and contained cholesterol clefts (Figure 16G). The neck specimen displayed matted lymph nodes adjacent to the jugular vein, that were up to 4 cm in diameter, and contained focally yellow, necrotic areas. The nodes exhibited squamous cell carcinoma, as shown in the needle biopsy specimen (Figure 16F). In summary, the patient had two lesions: (1) a Warthin's tumor of the parotid gland, and (2) a metastatic squamous cell carcinoma of the neck from an unknown primary tumor.

The patient developed supraclavicular, mediastinal, and pulmonary metastases that were treated with radiation therapy. He died ten months after his initial visit.

Comments

The CT sialogram demonstrated a mass in the right parotid gland. CT sialography is no longer utilized, since the majority of parotid lesions are well contrasted against the low attenuation glands.

The CT examination of the neck outlined an irregular mass of mixed attenuation, which obliterated the adjacent structures. The appearance was suggestive of metastatic, matted necrotic lymph nodes. In a patient of this age with a necrotic neck mass, metastatic squamous cell carcinoma was the most likley diagnosis. Lymph nodes, involved by lymphoma, rarely show necrosis (except occasionally, Hodgkin or histiocytic lymphomas).

In this case, MRI suggested that the Warthin's tumor was predominantly cystic [36], as evidenced by high SI on T_2-CW images. On Figure 16C, the deep neck mass had signal characteristics that were different from the parotid mass. Although, in this case, two histological entities were present (Warthin's tumor and squamous cell carcinoma), the signal characteristics alone do not justify the correct diagnosis of two lesions. One has to keep in mind that a single tumor may have a spectrum of different signal characteristics depending on the histologic composition of the tumor. This variability of MR signal characteristics (in the same tumor) is further highlighted in the next case.

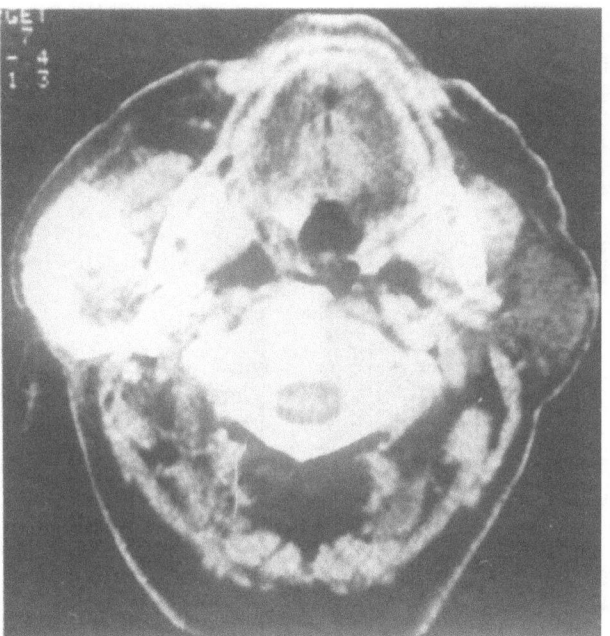

A

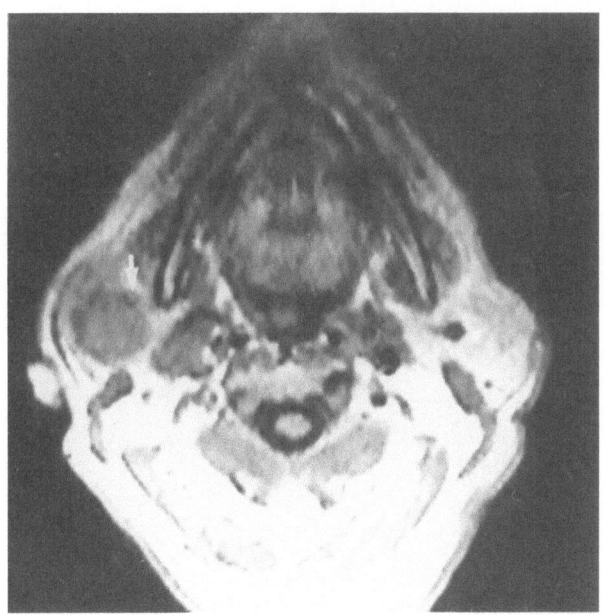

B

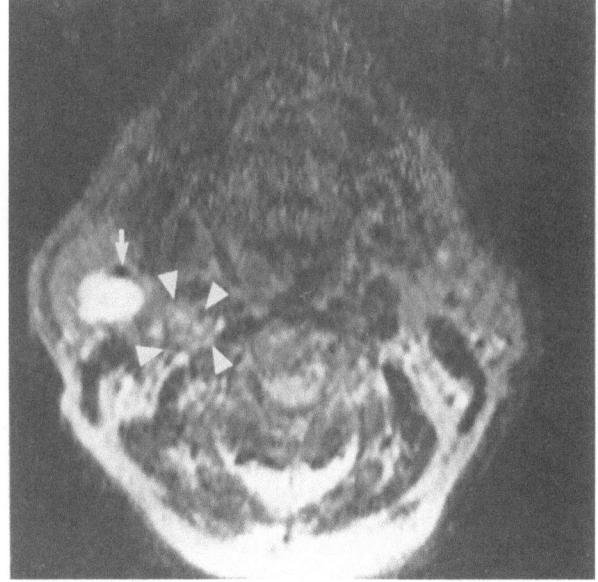

C

Figure 16.(A) *CT sialogram with axial section through the mid parotid glands* reveals a sharply defined, oval-shaped filling defect secondary to a right intraparotid mass.
(B & C) *Axial MR projections through the mid to lower parotid glands* [(17B) *TR* 500/*TE* 20 − NEX = 6; (17C) *TR* 2000/*TE* 96 − NEX = 4. SLT = 0.5 cm] demonstrate a well defined mass, with intermediate and high SI on the T_1- and T_2-CW images (Figures 16B & C) within the right parotid gland, adjacent to the posterior aspect of the RMV (arrow). The long *TE* (96 msec) results in greater loss of signal within the RMV on the T_2-CW image (Figure 16C) compared to the short *TE* (20 msec) on the T_1-CW image (Figure 16B). The T_2-CW image also demonstrates an ill-defined area (arrowheads) of relatively high SI in the deep neck, which is not evident on the T_1-CW image. This represents the carcinoma illustrated in Figures 16D & E.

D. Salivary glands

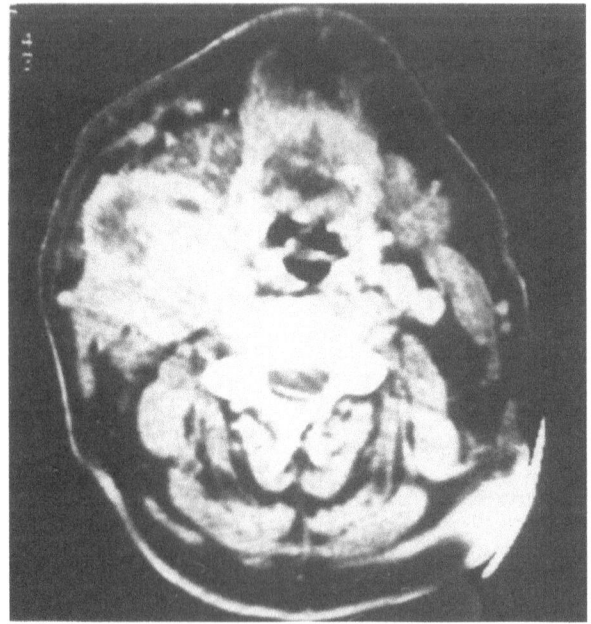

D

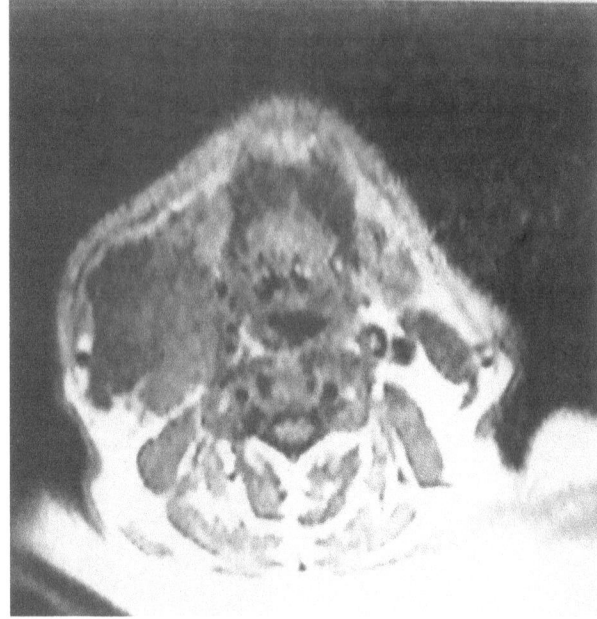

E

Figure 16.(D) *Contrast CT with axial section through the neck slightly above the hyoid bone* shows a large mixed density mass measuring about 5 cm in diameter. The appearance is consistent with matted, partially necrotic lymph nodes. The tumor compresses the posterior surface of the right submandibular gland which is displaced anteriorly. The fat plane between the mass and the sternocleidomastoid muscle, as well as the neurovascular sheath, are obliterated.

(E) *Axial MR projection at a comparable level* (*TR* 500/*TE* 20 − NEX = 6; SLT = 0.5 cm) demonstrates a lobulated mass of intermediate SI invading the sternocleidomastoid muscle posteriorly. There is obliteration of the fat surrounding the neurovascular bundle. This mass, on the T_2-CW image (not illustrated) reveals intermediate SI with bright areas corresponding to the suspected areas of necrosis on CT.

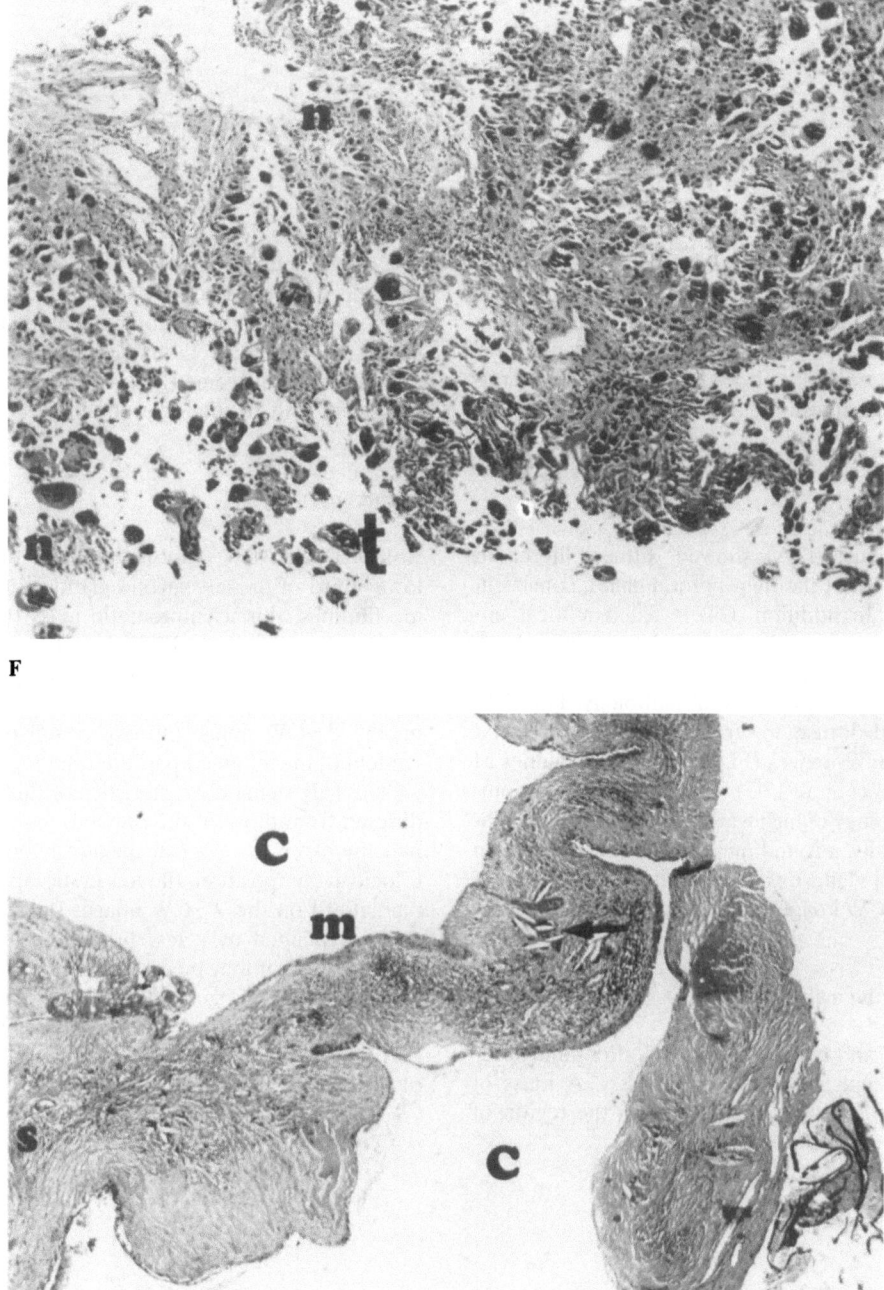

F

G

Figure 16.(F) *Photomicrograph of needle biopsy material taken from the neck mass* (79×, hematoxylin and eosin stain) shows squamous cell carcinoma with cellular polymorphism. Note tumor giant cells (t) and focal cell necrosis (n).

(G) *Photomicrograph of adenolymphoma of parotid gland* (31×, hematoxylin and eosin stain) with large, cystic spaces (C), flattened mucosa (m), fibrous stroma (s), and cholesterol clefts (arrow). Note absence of lymphoid cells.

D. Salivary glands

Case 17

WARTHIN'S TUMOR OF THE LEFT PAROTID GLAND

Clinical presentation

A 55 year old male complained of sudden swelling of the right parotid gland, consistent with a nonspecific parotitis. This swelling subsequently cleared, but the patient continued to experience intermittent, vague discomfort.

Radiologic findings

A CT study (Figure 17A) showed diffuse, increased attenuation throughout the right parotid gland, consistent with sialadenitis. In addition, CT revealed a focal enhancing mass in the lower third of the left parotid gland, which was clinically asymptomatic.

MRI also demonstrated bilateral pathology. The right parotid gland had diffuse, lower SI than the left parotid gland on the T_1-CW images (Figure 17D), and higher SI on T_2-CW images (Figure 17C). The T_2-CW SI was compatible with pathology of high water content, such as sialadenitis. Additionally, a round mass in the inferior portion of the left parotid gland displayed an intermediate SI on both T_1- and T_2-CW images (Figures 17B & C).

Surgical and histological findings

Based on the CT and MRI findings, and after clinical re-examination, the patient underwent surgery. A mass of approximately 1.5 cm was encountered in the region of the ramus mandibularis of the facial nerve and a left superficial parotidectomy was performed.

Histologically, the tumor was characterized by double layers of oxyphilic cells in papillary projections, folding into a lymphoid stroma (Figure 17E). These features were consistent with an adenolymphoma or Warthin's tumor.

Comments

Both CT and MRI, demonstrated the tumor mass in the lower third of the left parotid gland. Without these imaging findings, this asymptomatic mass (the patient never had any complaint) would not have been detected.

The sialadenitis in the right parotid gland is characterized on CT by increased density, and on MRI by a high SI on the T_2-CW image (an expression of the high water content of the inflamed parotid tissue). .

The MR signal characteristics of this Warthin's tumor differed from those of the previous case (Case 16), which had the same histological diagnosis, but a different histological composition (larger cystic spaces). The intermediate SI on the T_2-CW images (versus high SI in case 16) is explained by a less prominent cystic component. Warthin's tumor may be cystic or semisolid [36]. There are variations in the size and crystallization of cholesterol, and in the size of the cystic spaces in Warthin's tumors [37]. This histologic variation between cases 16 and 17 explains the different signal characteristics.

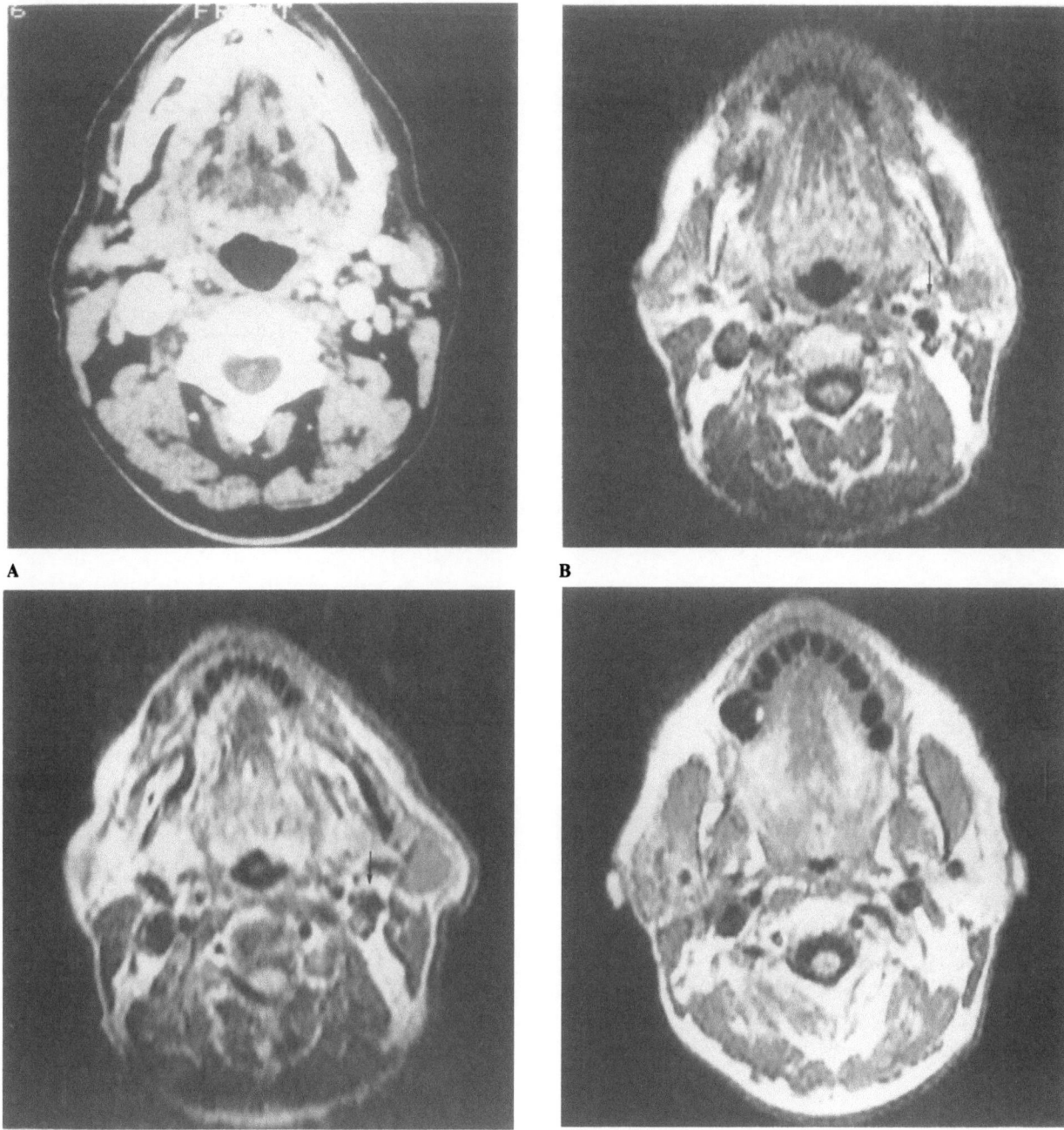

A

B

C

D

Figure 17.(A) *Axial contrast CT section through the lower third (tail) of the left parotid gland* shows a well demarcated, round, 1 cm mass. The right parotid gland has diffuse increased attenuation (also documented on other sections through the parotid gland that are not illustrated here). There is a small lymph node anterior to the internal jugular vein and medial to the left parotid gland, which measures 5–6 mm in diameter, and probably represents a small reactive lymph node of no significance.

(B & C) *Axial MR projections at a comparable level.* [(17B) *TR* 500/*TE* 20 − NEX = 6; (17C) *TR* 2000/*TE* 48 − NEX = 4. SLT = 0.5 cm] demonstrate a round mass in the lower third of the left parotid gland, adjacent to the retromandibular vein. The lesion

has intermediate to low SI on the T_1-CW image (Figure 17B) and on the mildly T_2-CW image (Figure 17C). An arrow points to a small lymph node anterior to the left internal jugular vein.

(D) *Axial MR projection at a more cephalad level* (same machine parameters as Figure 17B) demonstrates marked asymmetry in SI between the left and right parotid glands. The left parotid gland has on this T_1-CW image, normal relatively high SI (intermediate between fat and muscle), while the right parotid gland has a diffusely, lower SI, consistent with either fibrosis and/or inflammation. The T_2-CW images (not illustrated) show high SI within the right parotid gland, indicating high water content and therefore, inflammation.

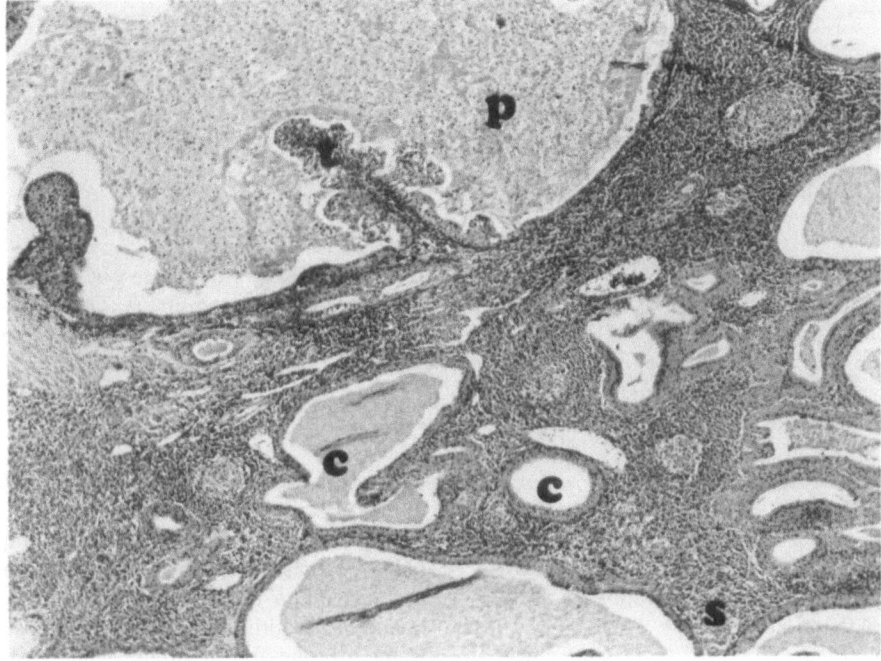

E

Figure 17.(E) *Photomicrograph of adenolymphoma of the parotid gland after superficial parotidectomy* (50×, hematoxylin and eosin stain) shows the tumor with papillary projections (t), small, cystic spaces (c) with protein debris (p) and lymphoid stroma (s).

Case 18

ONCOCYTOMA OF THE LEFT PAROTID GLAND

Clinical presentation

A 40 year old woman presented with a left upper neck mass. On examination, the mass was firm and localized to the left parotid gland, without facial nerve weakness. There were no palpable nodes in the neck.

Radiologic findings

A contrast CT study with axial sections (Figure 18A) showed an oval lesion in the superficial lobe of the left parotid gland lateral to the RMV.

MRI, with axial (Figures 18B, C, & D) and coronal (Figure 18E & F) projections revealed an ill-defined mass within the superficial lobe of the left parotid gland lateral to the RMV. No neck lymph nodes were identified. This lesion was of intermediate SI on both the T_1- and T_2-CW images with little contrast with the normal gland.

Surgical and histopathological findings

At surgery, the mass was adjacent to the RMV and deviated the facial nerve medially (which anatomically is lateral to the RMV). A left superficial parotidectomy was performed and a transitory facial paresis developed postoperatively.

Pathological specimens from sections through the excised parotid tissue (Figure 18G) showed replacement and distortion of the superficial parotid gland by a tumor composed of large oxyphilic cells with abundant cytoplasms and small, round, regular nuclei (Figure 18H).

Duct structures were not present in the tumor region, and there was only scant fibrosis. These histological findings were characteristics of an oncocytoma [38].

Comments

The lesion was well demonstrated on CT, whereas the tumor was not clearly depicted on the T_1- and T_2-CW MR images. MR image contrast was improved using the phase contrast technique [32, 39]. This technique results in cancellation of the RF signals of fat and water contained in parotid tissue. Tissues composed of all fat or all water protons appear bright, while tissues with both fat and water protons, such as bone marrow or parotid gland, appear dark. The effect of this technique is manifested by a dark parotid gland and a lesion of possibly high SI contrasted against the low SI gland.

However, MR showed the lesion in closer proximity to the RMV, and by inference to the facial nerve, than suggested by CT. This was confirmed at surgery. The relationship of the tumor to the facial nerve is important in the surgical planning, and MRI permits direct imaging of the facial nerve on thin-section MR images, using surface coils [34].

This particular case, with a histological diagnosis of oncocytoma, did not display the typical MR signal characteristics of parotid neoplasms, with high SI on the T_2-CW images [31]. Pleomorphic adneomas, which represent 85% of parotid tumors, usually have a high SI on the T_2-CW images, which is probably related to the large amount of myxoid stroma.

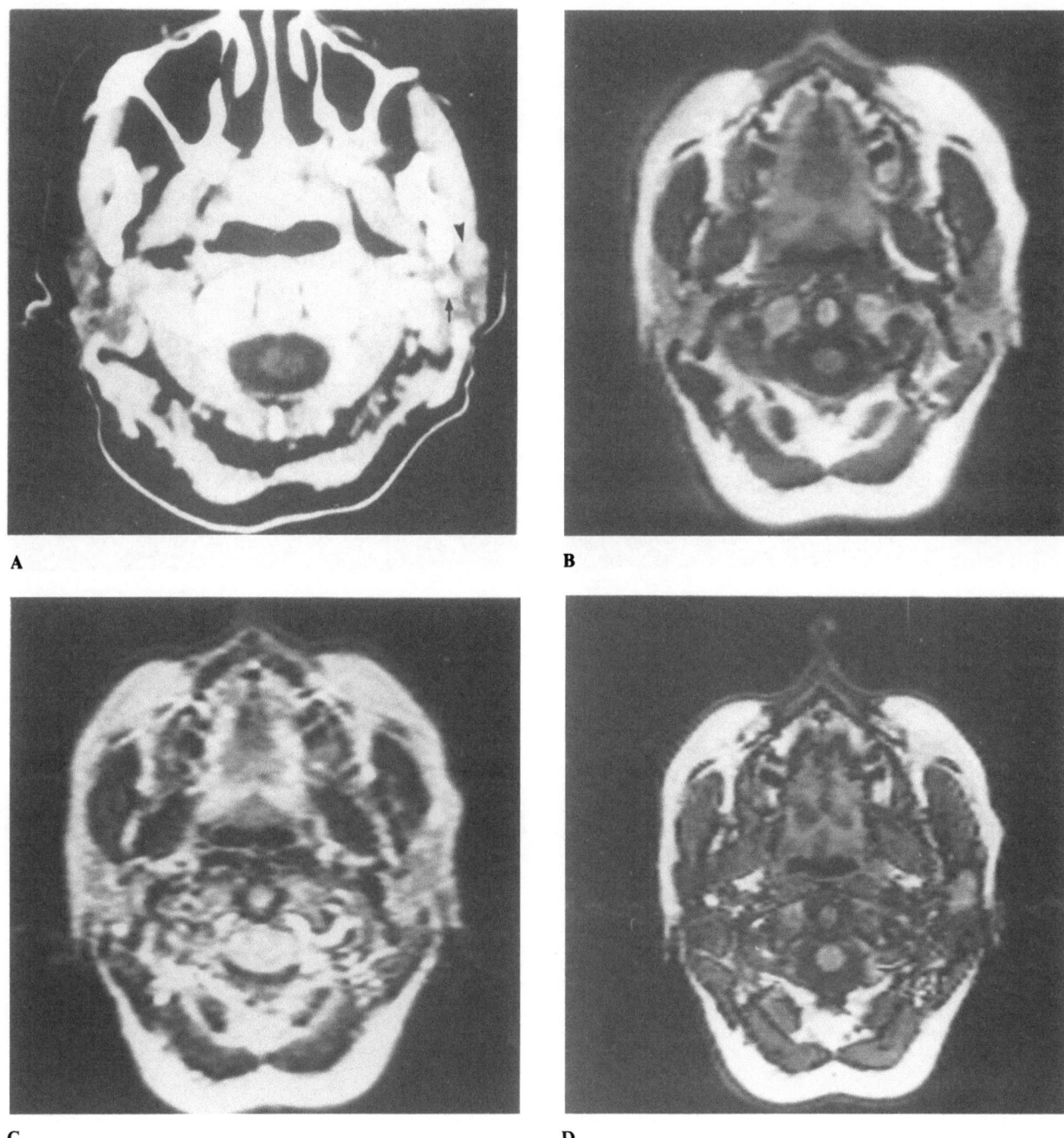

A

B

C

D

Figure 18.(A) *Axial contrast CT section through the parotid glands* outlines a round, slightly lobulated, homogeneous, well demarcated lesion in the lower third of the left parotid gland adjacent to the posterior masseter muscle (arrowhead). An enhancing structure, medial and posterior to the lesion represents the RMV (arrow).
(B & C) *Axial MR projections at a comparable level* [(18C) *TR* 400/*TE* 20 − NEX = 4; (18D) *TR* 2000/*TE* 96 − NEX = 2. SLT = 0.5 cm] demonstrate an ill-defined area of intermediate SI within the anterior portion of the superficial lobe of the left paro-

tid gland, which is better delineated on the T_1-CW image (Figure 18B). The SI is slightly lower than normal parotid tissue on both the T_1-CW (Figure 18B) and the T_2-CW (Figure 18C) images, and therefore, is not optimally shown.
(D) *Axial MR 'chemical shift image' at a similar level* (*TR* 300/ *TE* 20 − NEX = 4; SLT = 0.5 cm) demonstrates low SI of the normal parotid gland due to the cancellation effect of signal contributions from fat and water protons. On this low SI background, the intraparotid lesion, which has little fat content, exhibits high SI.

D. Salivary glands

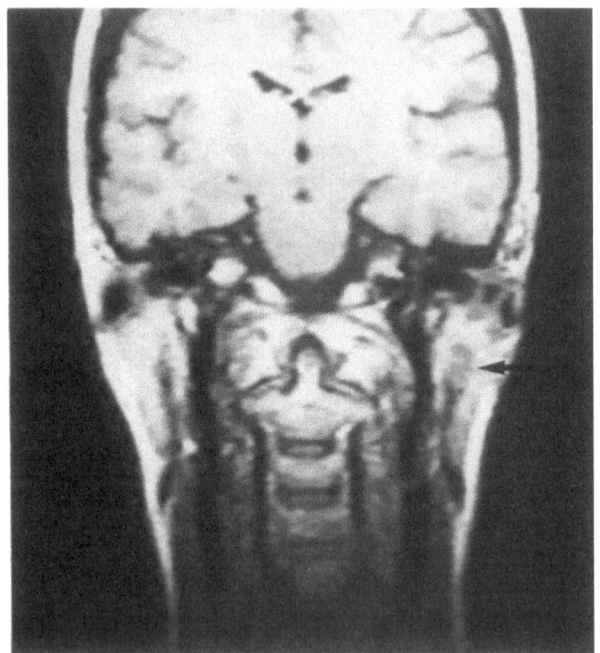 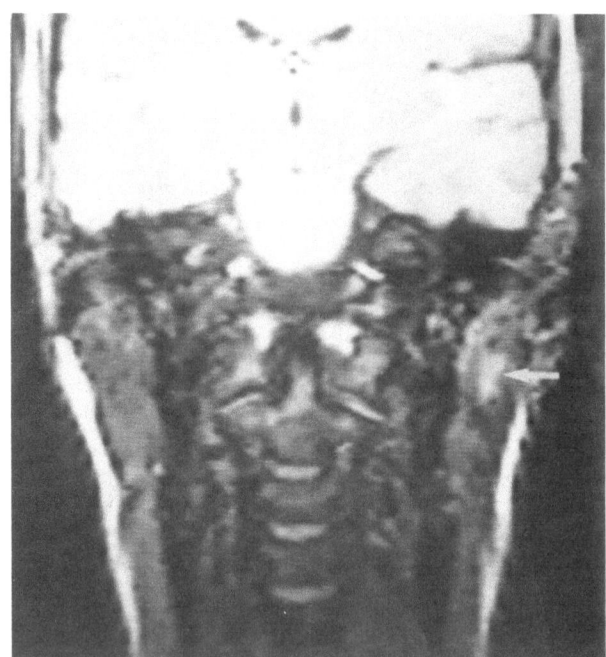

E   F

Figure 18.(E) *Coronal MR projection (TR* 400/*TE* 20 − NEX = 4; SLT = 0.4 cm) through the posterior aspect of the mass confirms the presence of an ill-defined lesion, of intermediate SI (arrow).
(F) *Comparable MR coronal 'chemical shift image' (TR* 300/*TE* 25 − NEX = 4; SLT = 0.7 cm) demonstrates low SI within normal parotid gland and vertebral bone marrow due to the cancellation effect of signal contributions from fat and water protons. There is high SI in the intraparotid lesion (arrow). Note also the high SI in predominantly water containing intervertebral discs and the high fat containing subcutaneous tissue.

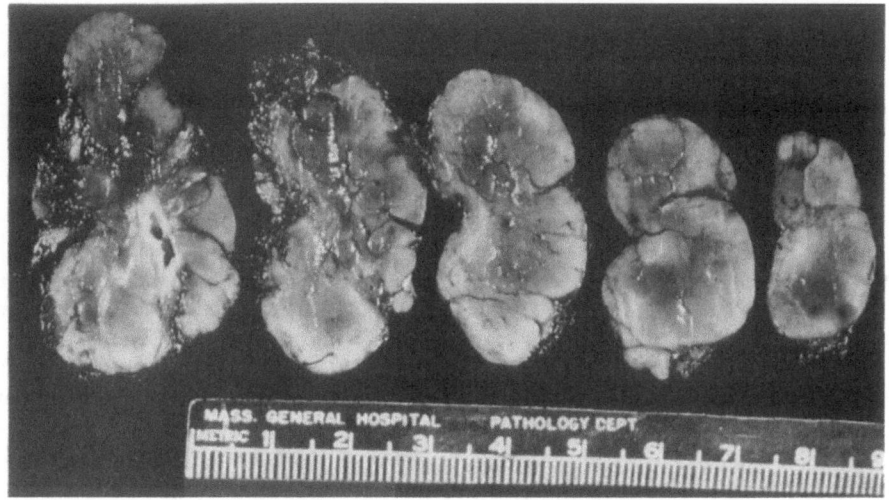

G

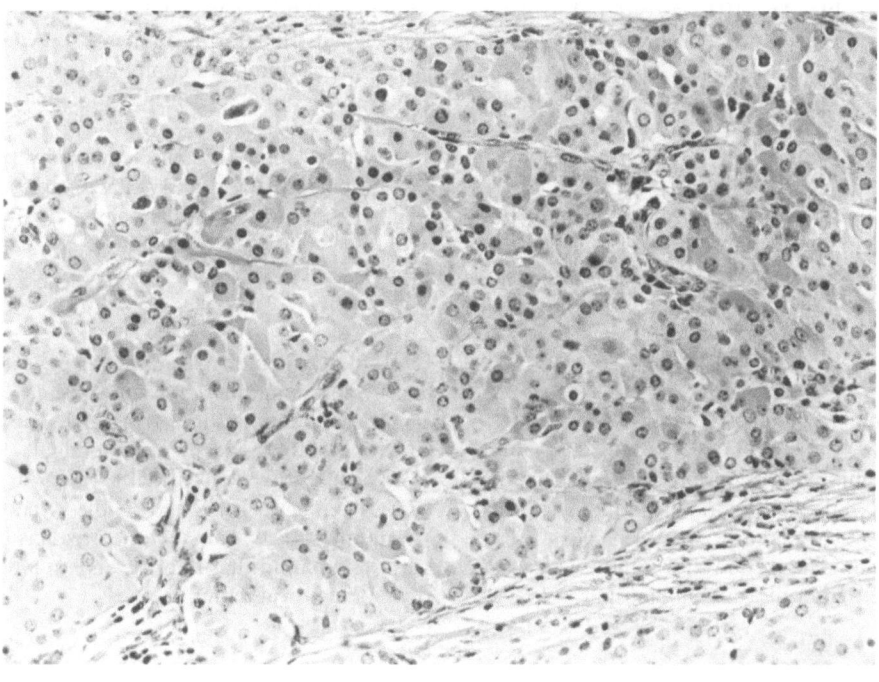

H

Figure 18.(G) *Multiple cross sections through the parotid gland after partial fixation.* The paler areas, at the periphery, are fixed normal parotid tissue, and the central, darker areas are oxyphilic tumor replacing parotid parenchyma.

(H) *Photomicrograph of parotid oncocytoma* (200×, hematoxylin and eosin stain) shows rounded, ovoid cells in nests and clusters. Note abundant cellular cytoplasm with small, round, regular nuclei.

Case 19

FOCAL CARCINOMA IN PLEOMORPHIC ADENOMA
OF THE LEFT PAROTID GLAND

Clinical presentation

A 64 year old man presented with a one and one-half year history of a left preauricular mass, which had been increasing in size for about nine months, without any other symptomatology. There was no past history of a scalp tumor.

Physical examination revealed a hard, mobile, nontender, 2 cm mass in the left preauricular area, probably within the parotid gland. The ENT examination was otherwise unremarkable. An MRI was ordered to determine the location of the lesion in relation to the parotid gland.

Radiologic findings

An MRI, with axial and coronal projections, demonstrated a well delineated, 2 cm mass, confined to the superior part of the superficial portion of the left parotid gland (Figures 19A & B). On the T_2-CW images, this tumor had heterogeneous signal characteristics (Figure 19C).

Surgical and pathological findings

At surgery, a multilobulated tumor was found in the superficial portion of the left parotid gland that was easily dissected free from the superior branch of the facial nerve.

Pathological examination showed a tumor, which was sharply demarcated from the surrounding parotid tissue (Figure 19D), and composed of dense fibrous tissue, myxoid tissue, ductal structures, and microcystic areas filled with proteinaceous debris. These histological features were consistent with a pleomorphic adenoma. However, in the central part of the tumor, there was a necrotic area with hemorrhage and cholesterol deposits (Figure 19E). In focal areas, the tumor showed hyperchromatic nuclei with nuclear cytoplasmic ratio alterations, indicative of malignancy. There were also focal infiltrative patterns that extended to normal parotid tissue. All of these combined findings were felt to warrant a diagnosis of carcinoma in pleomorphic adenoma. Additionally, fibrous tissue was a dominant component of the tumor, in several areas, as is often seen in pleomorphic adenomas of long duration.

Postoperative irradiation was delivered to the parotid area. The patient is doing well with no evidence of disease, eighteen months after treatment.

Comments

MRI clearly demonstrated the intraparotid location of the mass, differentiating between a preauricular lymph node and parotid tumor. Moreover, MRI showed the absence of invasion of the adjacent, peripheral fat.

The heterogeneous SI of the tumor mass, mainly on the T_2-CW images, is related to the varied histologic composition. The central, necrotic area has high SI, while the rest of the tumor has intermediate to low SI, reflecting the extensive fibrous component.

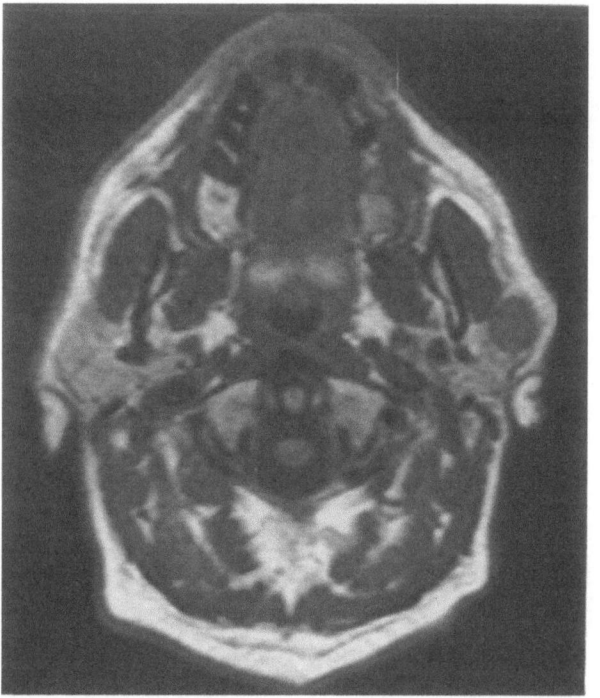

A

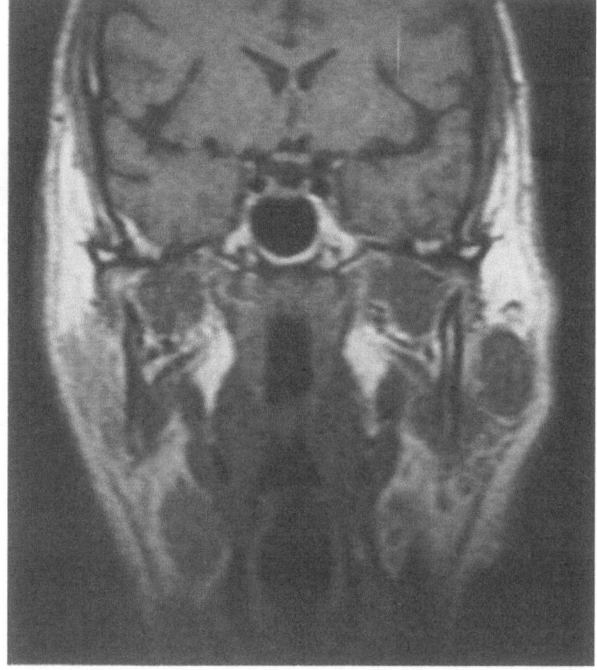

B

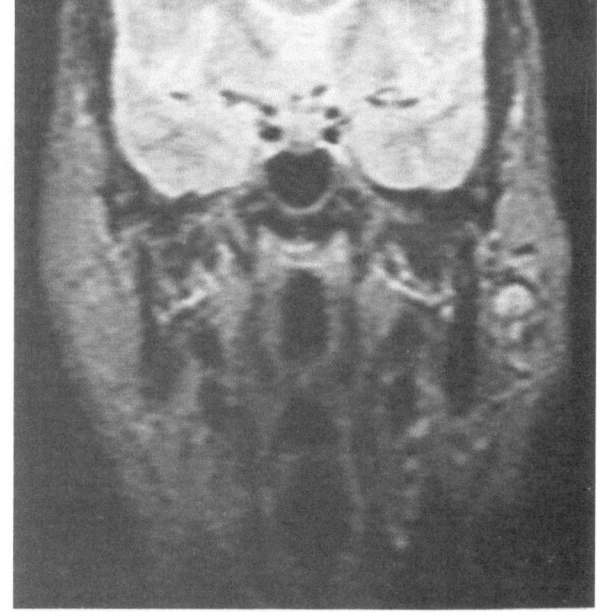

C

Figure 19.(A) *Axial MR image through mid parotid level (TR 450/TE 22 − NEX = 6; SLT = 0.5 cm)* shows a well defined mass of intermediate to low SI within the anterior aspect of the superficial portion of the left parotid gland.
(B & C) *Coronal MR images through the anterior aspect of the parotid glands* [(19B) *TR 450/TE 22 − NEX = 6; (19C) TR*

2000/*TE 96 − NEX = 2. SLT = 0.4 cm*] demonstrate a mass with intermediate to low SI on the T_1-CW image (Figure 19B) and heterogeneous SI on the T_2-CW image (Figure 19C). On Figure 19C, the superior third of the mass reveals high SI, while the inferior two thirds are heterogeneous with intermediate and high SI.

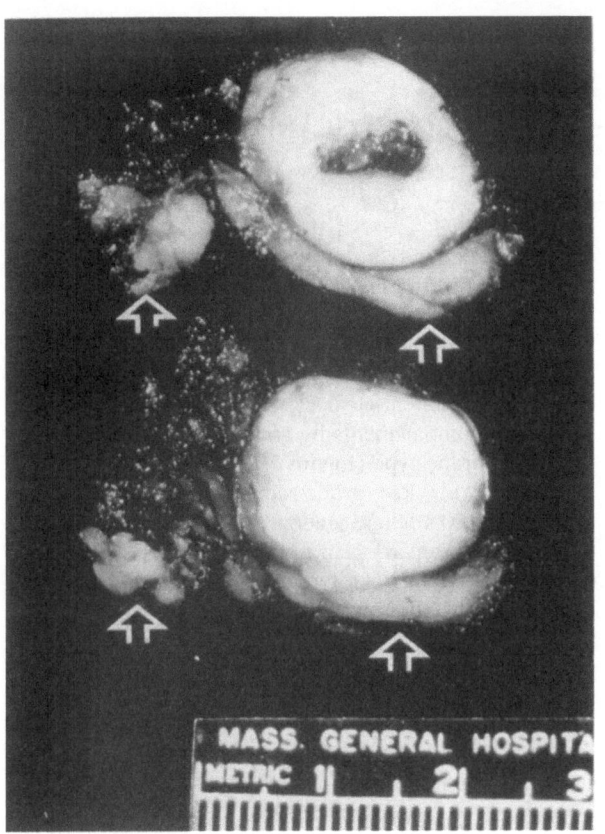

D

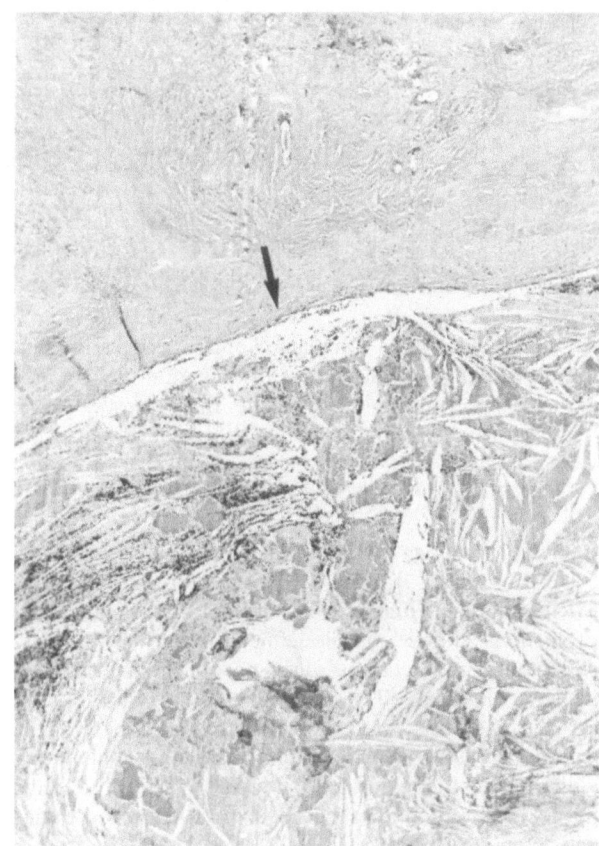

E

Figure 19.(D) *Photomicrograph of cut surfaces of the excised tumor mass (carcinoma in pleomorphic adenoma).* The lower specimen section shows a solid tumor. The upper specimen section shows tumor with central necrosis and cavitation. Note normal parotid tissue (arrows).

(E) *Photomicrograph of the excised specimen (carcinoma in pleomorphic adenoma)* (75×, hematoxylin and eosin stain) shows a cystic area with necrosis and multiple cholesterol clefts. These cholesterol clefts, in the prefixed specimen, are filled with cholesterol crystals. An arrow indicates the cyst wall.

Case 20

ADENOCARCINOMA OF THE RIGHT PAROTID GLAND

Clinical presentation

A 26 year old woman complained of right ear pain radiating down her jaw. On physical examination, there was a 1.5 cm mobile, firm mass in the right parotid gland. Neither facial weakness nor neck lymphadenopathies were noted.

Radiologic findings

MRI, with axial (Figure 20A) and coronal (Figure 20B) projections showed an ill-defined, right parotid mass within the superficial and deep portion, that had intermediate and high SI respectively, on T_1- and T_2-CW images. The mass extended to the inferior aspect of the external auditory canal. No abnormal lymph nodes were identified in the right neck. Because of the ill-defined borders, the differential diagnosis included mixed tumor and carcinoma.

Surgical and histological findings

At surgery, a mass primarily medial to the facial nerve, was peeled off the facial nerve branches and removed. There was no bony involvement. A near total parotidectomy with preservation of the facial nerve was carried out.

The excised parotid specimen contained a circumscribed tumor mass with nodular projections (Figure 20C) along with capsular and focal perineural infiltrations. There were also foci, suggestive of vascular invasion. Remaining tumor was present at the resection margins and in the facial nerve area. On histopathologic examination, the tumor consisted of lobules with minute, acinar structures. These structures were lined by cuboidal epithelial cells and surrounded by stratified myoepithelial cells with prominent clear cystoplasm. The cells were divided into compartments by connective tissue of a basement membrane type (Figure 20D). These findings were consistent with low grade adenocarcinoma. The cell morphology was heterogeneous with a predominant pattern of a rare salivary gland tumor called epithelial-myoepithelial carcinoma of intercalated duct origin [40].

Because of the possibility of residual disease, the patient received 60.8 Gy, delivered twice a day. The patient was without evidence of disease two years after surgery.

Comments

This type of tumor is rare and it has been questioned whether the lesion represents an adenoma or adenocarcinoma [40]. Histologically, this tumor had an infiltrative pattern, which correlated with the MR appearance of an irregular, intraparotid mass invading the fat, adjacent to the auditory canal. Furthermore, the lesion involved both the deep and superficial portions of the parotid gland. All of these morphological features suggested a malignant tumor. This tumor was imaged by MR, in the axial and coronal planes. Coronal sections are useful for assessing superior–inferior extension, cervical lymphadenopathy, and the base of the skull.

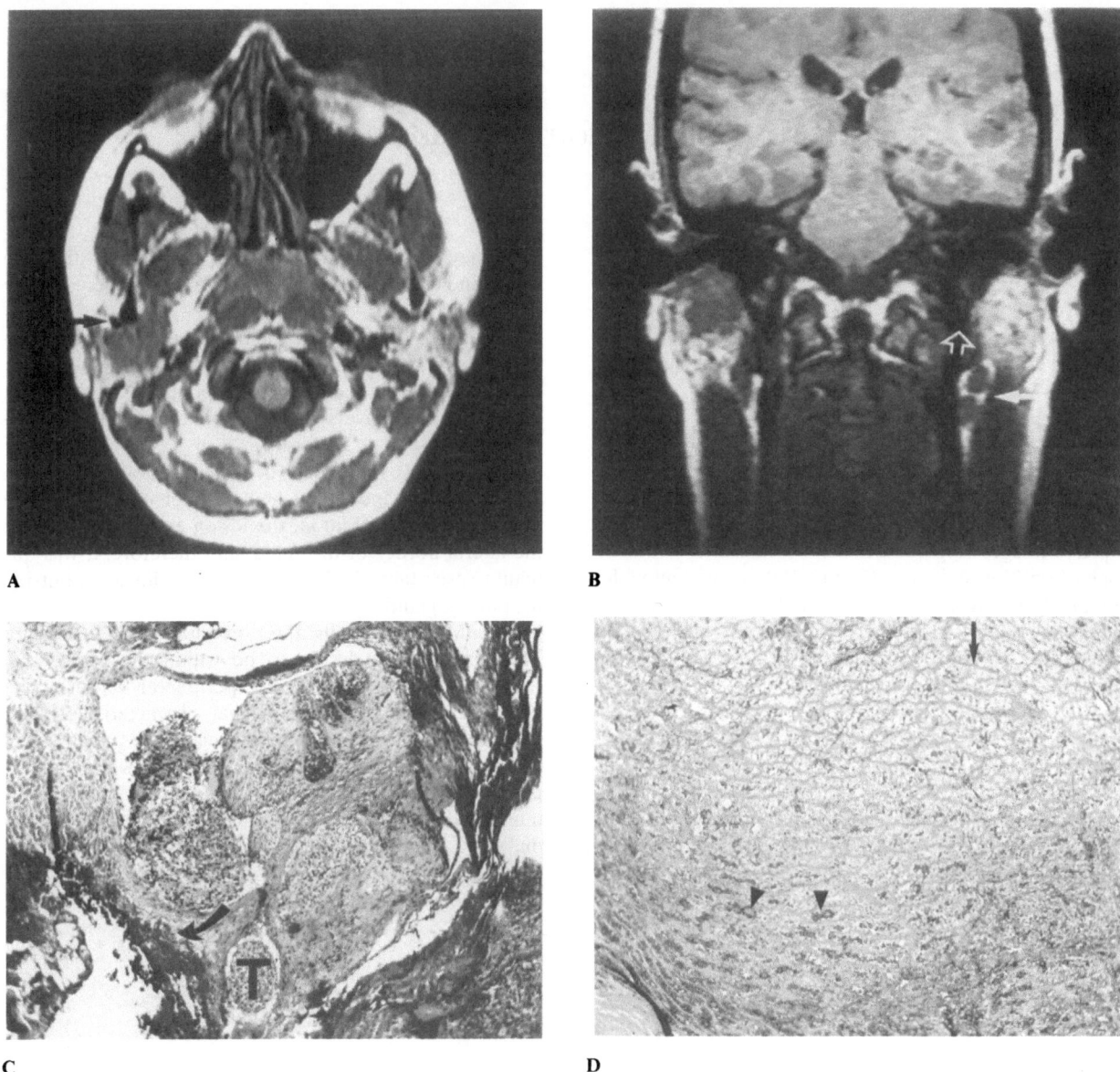

A

B

C

D

Figure 20. **(A)** *Axial MR projection through mid parotid gland* (*TR* 400/*TE* 21 − NEX = 6; SLT = 0.5 cm) reveals an ill-defined mass of intermediate SI within the superficial and deep portion of right parotid gland displacing RMV laterally (arrow).
(B) *Coronal MR projection through external auditory canal* (*TR* 400/*TE* 21 − NEX = 6; SLT = 0.4 cm) demonstrates an irregular mass of intermediate SI within the right parotid gland, extending to the external auditory canal. Note two jugulodigastric lymph nodes (1 cm in size) on the left side (arrow), and jugular vein (open arrow).

(C) *Photomicrograph of a section through the excised parotid specimen* (55×, hematoxylin and eosin stain) shows an epithe-lial-myoepithelial carcinoma with tumor nodules (T) and cap-sular infiltration (arrow).
(D) *Photomicrograph of epithelial-myoepithelial carcinoma* (55×, hematoxylin eosin stain) shows septation of the tumor (arrow) with central epithelial acini (arrowheads).

Case 21

LIPOMA OF THE RIGHT PAROTID GLAND

Clinical presentation

A 27 year old woman presented with a nontender, rubber-like mass located over the angle of the right mandible. The physical examination was otherwise unremarkable.

Radiographic findings

The initial CT contrast study was interpreted as normal. An MR examination demonstrated a mass of high SI on T_1-CW images (Figures 21A & C), and intermediate – high SI on T_2-CW images (Figure 21B), consistent with a lipoma. In retrospect, the CT study also showed the parotid lipoma (Figure 21D). Because of the minimal cosmetic deformity and the potential danger of surgery in this area, it was decided to follow the patient.

Comments

Lipomas of the parotid gland are rare tumors, but arise, most often, in the subcutaneous tissue of the neck [41–42]. They may be located at the margin or within the gland, and cause a filling defect or localized indentation of the parotid tissue.

Lipomas are usually well defined, but occasionally extend along the fascial planes into the adjacent tissues. Fibrous septae are found in large lipomatous masses and, on CT, lipomas have a characteristic low attenuation coefficient.

On CT, this lesion was not well separated from the adjacent subcutaneous fat and was not detected by the first observer. In addition, the lesion appeared to indent the lateral border of the gland, and therefore, it was difficult to ascertain whether the lesion was inside or outside the parotid gland.

The MRI, especially the coronal projection (Figure 21C), showed the lesion to be within the gland, surrounded by the low intensity peripheral capsule. The mass-like appearance and signal characteristics were pathognomonic of a lipoma. Lipomas have a high signal intensity on T_1- and T_2-CW images. MRI, with its multiplanar capability and superior contrast resolution facilitates the definition, characterization, and location of lipomas.

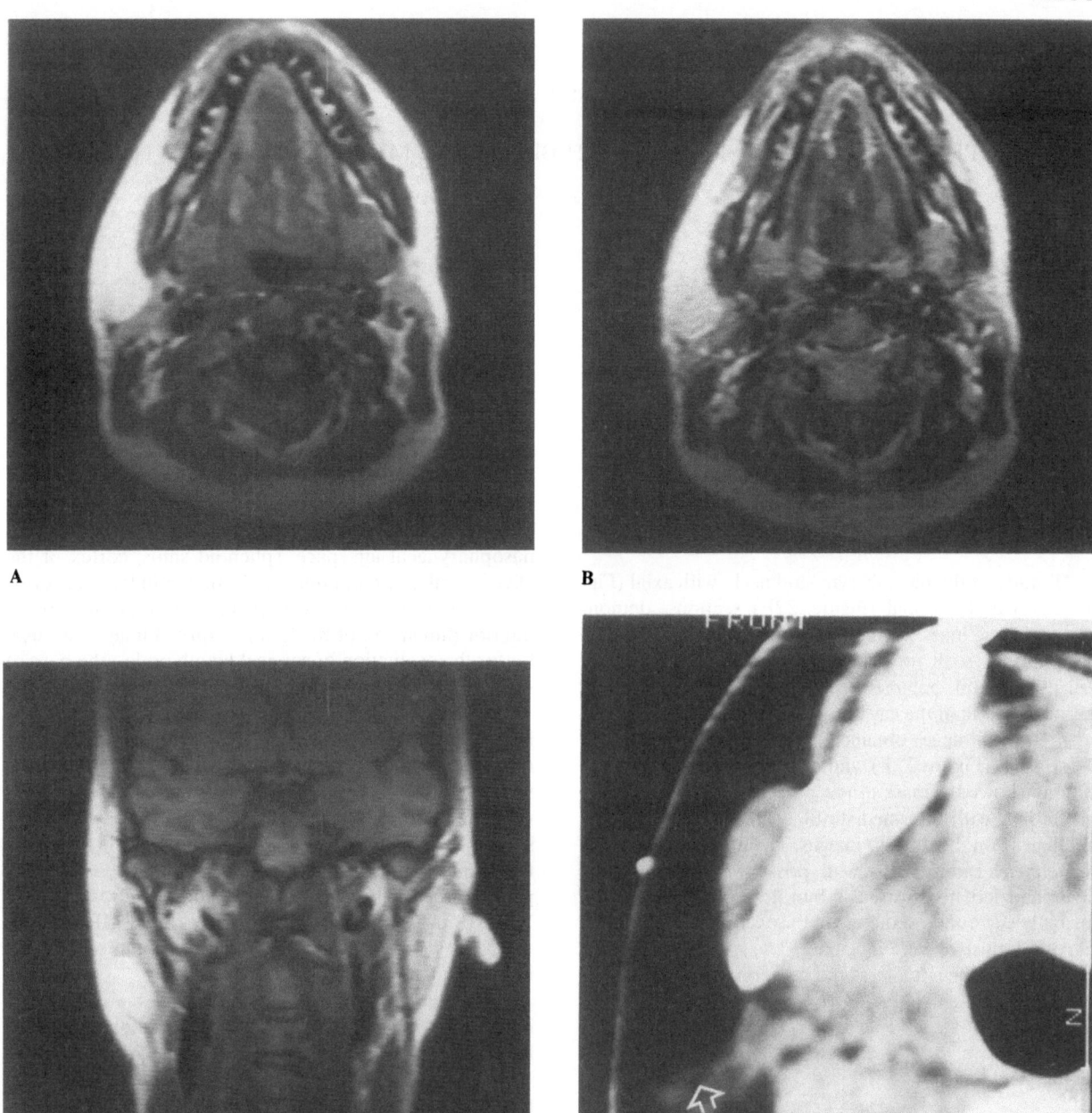

A

B

C

D

Figures 21.(A & B) *Axial MR projections* [(21A) *TR 500/TE 21 − NEX = 4; (21B) TR 2000/TE 96 − NEX = 2. SLT = 0.5 cm*] demonstrate a sharply defined mass of high SI on T_1- (Figure 21A) and T_2-CW images (Figure 21B) in the anterolateral aspect of the right parotid gland. These signal characteristics are similar to those of the adjacent subcutaneous fat. Note the linear, low SI capsule at the lateral margin of the lesion on the T_1-CW image.
(C) *Coronal MR projection* (*TR 500/TE 21 − NEX = 4; SLT =*

0.5 cm) confirms the presence of the mass within the right parotid gland.
(D) *Axial contrast CT section through the lower right parotid gland* reveals a sharply marginated lesion (2−3 cm in greatest diameter) causing indentation (arrow) of the lateral lower right parotid gland. This lesion had low attenuation consistent with a lipoma, but poor contrast with the adjacent subcutaneous fat and parotid gland.

Case 22

NASOPHARYNGEAL CARCINOMA WITH BILATERAL METASTATIC LYMPH NODES

Clinical presentation

A 62 year old woman complained for one year of left nasal obstruction and bleeding, otalgia, and a feeling of a blocked ear. On clinical examination, there was a left middle ear effusion and bilateral cervical lymph nodes were palpated in the neck. A biopsy of the nasopharynx revealed a carcinoma. The tumor was staged as T3N2MO.

Radiologic findings

A CT study of the nasopharynx and neck, with axial (Figure 22A) and coronal (Figure 22E) sections, demonstrated a large mass within the central and left part of the nasopharynx, with no evidence of bone destruction, as well as bilateral, enlarged, cervical lymph nodes. There was no invasion of the cavernous sinus.

MRI, with images obtained in axial (Figures 22B, C & D), coronal (Figure 22F), and sagittal (Figure 22G) projections showed a mass in the nasopharynx, more bulky on the left, with intermediate SI on the T_1-CW images, and high SI on the T_2-CW images. The tumor was close to the left cavernous sinus, with possible invasion of the clivus and left neurovascular bundle. The tissue planes, normally surrounding the medial aspect of the left lateral pterygoid muscle, were indistinct. The mass extended inferiorly along the left lateral and posterior pharyngeal wall to the level of the palate.

Histological findings

A biopsy taken from the nasopharynx revealed tumor cells arranged in sheets and nests. These rounded, ovoid cells had vesicular nuclei, prominent nucleoli, and numerous mitoses. Lymph nodes were scattered among the nuclei and composed the stroma (Figure 22H). The features were consistent with an undifferentiated carcinoma of lymphoepitheliomatous type.

Comments

Although CT, in the coronal and axial planes, demonstrated the tumor in the nasopharynx. MR was superior to CT in determining the soft tissue extension of the tumor due to greater tissue contrast and its multiplanar capability [43]. Determination of soft tissue extension is necessary for accurate designation of the radiation field [44]. The parapharyngeal space, including the lateral and medial pterygoid muscles, is better evaluated on the axial and coronal MR images. The sagittal views outline the nasopharyngeal air space, sphenoid sinus, cortex of the clivus, sella, prepontine and premedullary cisternal spaces, and upper cervical spine, as well as the superoinferior dimension of the lesion. Coronal images are useful for the evaluation of cervical lymph nodes, the base of skull, and cavernous sinus.

Although both modalities demonstrated bilateral, enlarged, cervical lymph nodes, the contour of these neck nodes is better defined on MR, particularly their interface with the adjacent muscles and the posterior margin of the submandibular glands. Both T_1- and T_2-CW images should be obtained. The T_1-CW images provide the high fat-lymph node contrast (Figure 22B) and T_2-CW images provide the high muscle-lymph node contrast (Figure 22C). Both CT (low attenuation areas) and MR (high SI on T_2-CW images) indicated necrosis, commonly found in large squamous cell metastases.

The high SI of the nasopharyngeal tissue on T_2-CW images is consistent with the histological finding of a very lymphoid stroma without fibrosis.

Design of the MRI exam must take into account the primary nasopharyngeal tumor and the lymph node chains, which drain the nasopharynx. Axial, coronal, and sagittal images should be obtained with inclusion of the upper and mid neck (including the jugulodigastric lymph node drainage area). If metastatic nodes are observed in the upper neck, an additional axial examination of the remaing neck and upper mediastinum should follow, and include T_1- and T_2-CW images.

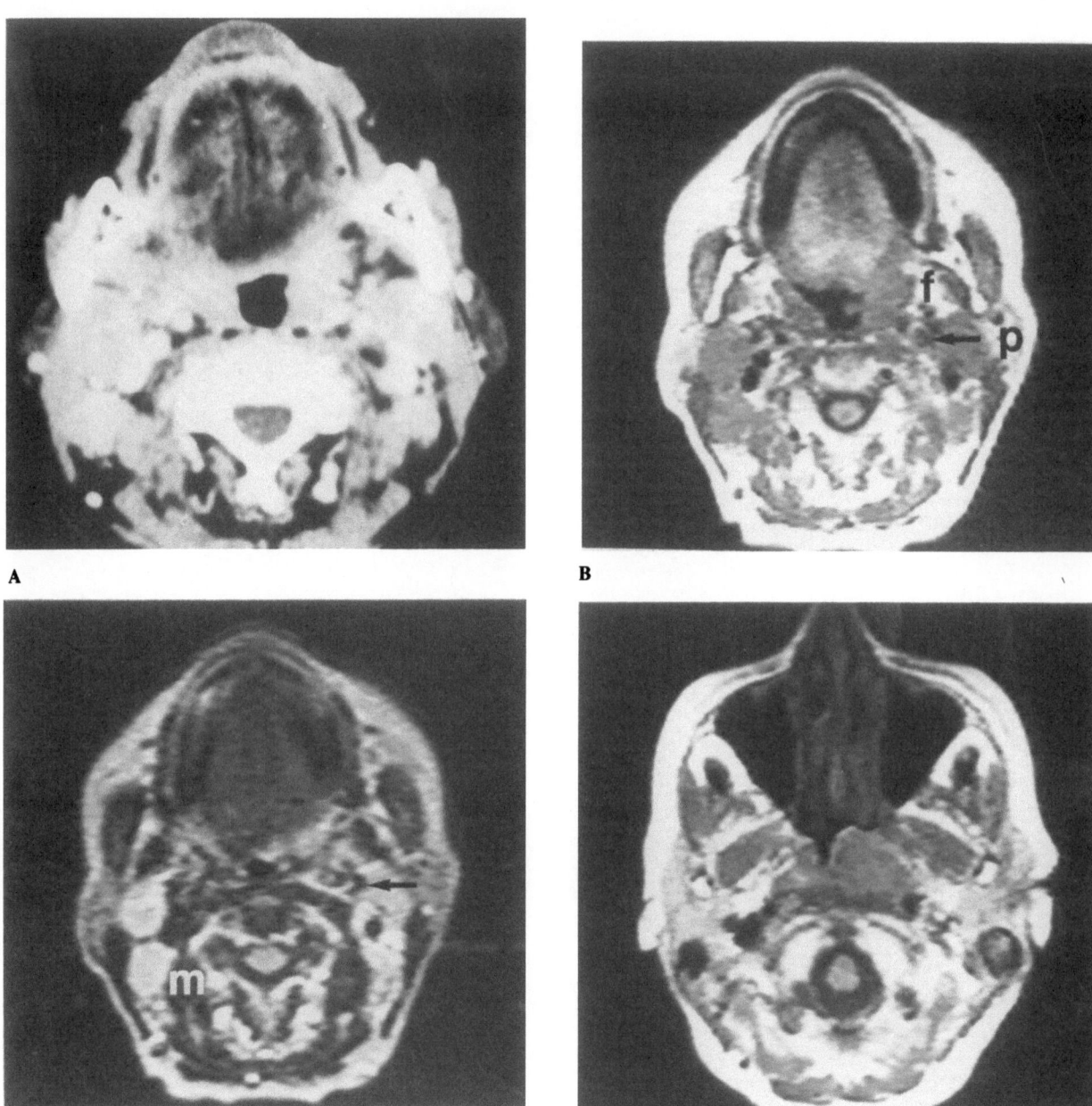

A

B

C

D

Figure 22.(A) *Axial contrast CT section slightly above the angle of the mandible* reveals matted lymph nodes, adjacent to the right vascular sheath, and in the right posterior triangle. On the left, there is a 2 cm node anterior and lateral to the vascular sheath, and a 1.5 cm node in the posterior triangle adjacent to the vascular sheath.
(B & C) *Comparable axial MR projections* [(22B) *TR* 500/*TE* 20 − NEX = 4; (22C) *TR* 2000/*TE* 96 − NEX = 2. SLT = 0.7 cm]. The lymph nodes have intermediate SI on the T_1-CW image (Figure 22B) and high SI on the T_2-CW image (Figure 22C). Contrast of lymph nodes with fat (f) and with parotid glands (p) is better shown on the T_1-CW image, while contrast of lymph nodes with muscle (m) is better defined on the T_2-CW image.

Note the separation of the internal carotid artery (arrow) from the internal jugular vein on the left by the lymph nodes.
(D) *Axial MR projection at level of nasopharynx* (*TR* 500/*TE* 20 − NEX = 4; SLT = 0.7 cm). A mass of intermediate SI is seen in the nasopharynx, in close apposition to the posterior edge of the left inferior turbinate. Posteriorly, the mass invades the longus colli and capitis muscles and the fat plane medial to the left, lateral pterygoid muscle. The mass approximates both internal carotid arteries, but does not encase them. The left mastoid air cells reveal intermediate to high SI on this T_1-CW image and high SI on T_2-CW image (not shown), compatible with retained mucoid fluid.

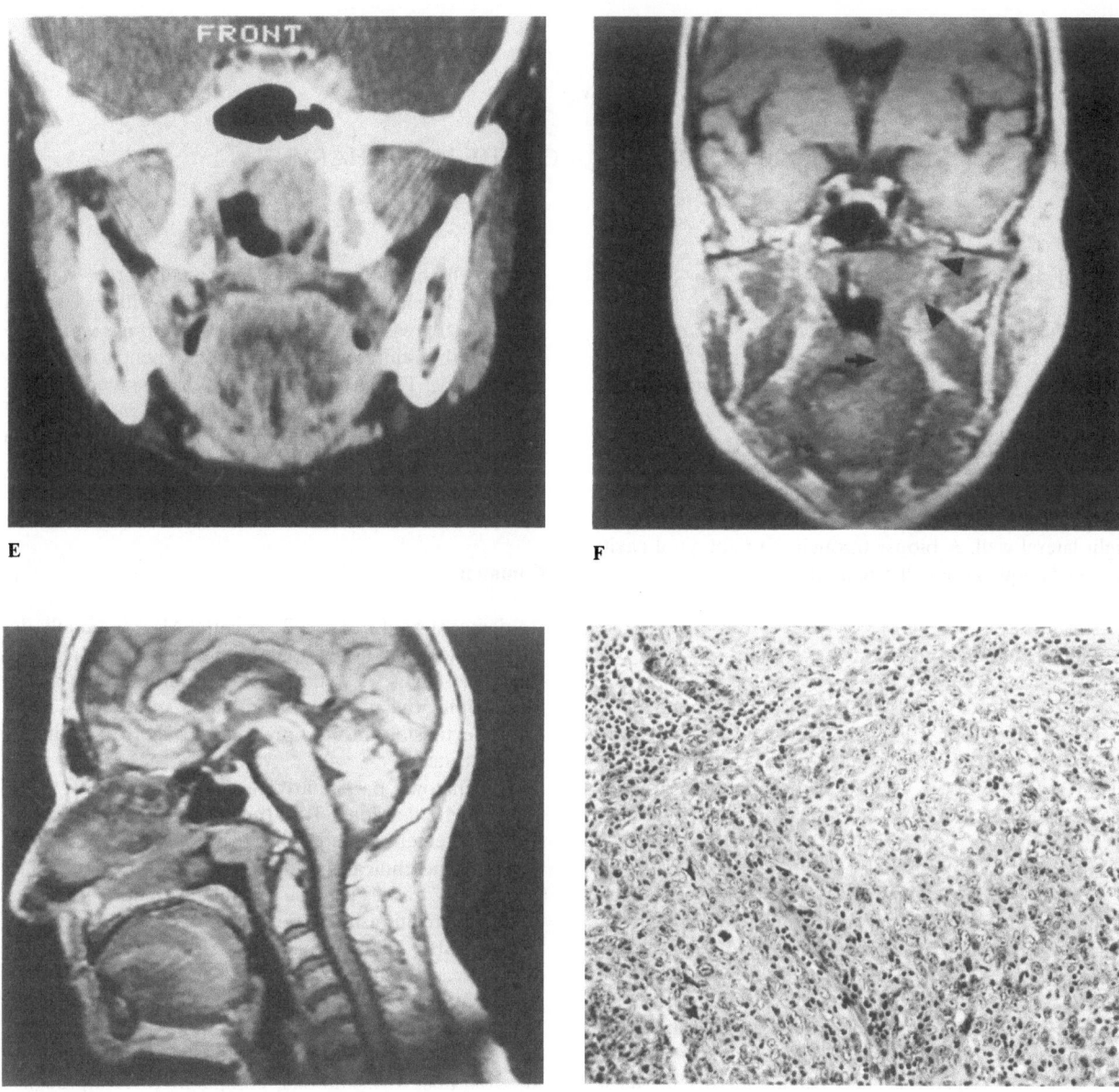

E

F

G

H

Figure 22. (E) *Coronal contrast CT section through the naso-pharynx* reveals a homogeneous mass in the central and left portion of the nasopharynx, without bone destruction.
(F) *Coronal MR projection* (*TR* 500/*TE* 20 − NEX = 4; SLT = 0.7 cm). The mass of intermediate SI fills both sides of the nasopharynx and does not invade the sphenoid sinus. It is uncertain whether there is invasion of the cavernous sinus. On the left side, the fatty planes surrounding the pterygoid muscles are indistinct (arrowheads). The mass extends inferiorly along the left lateral pharyngeal wall to the level of the uvula (arrow).

(G) *Sagittal MR projection* (*TR* 500/*TE* 20 − NEX = 4; SLT = 0.7 cm). The tumor fills the upper part of the nasopharynx, is close to the choanae anteriorly, and the basisphenoid superiorly. The tumor infiltrates the posterior wall of the nasopharynx to the level of the soft palate. The marrow within the clivus, the C1 and C2 vertebral bodies, as well as their bony cortices, are normal.
(H) *Photomicrograph of a biopsy from the nasopharynx* shows undifferentiated carcinoma of lymphoepitheliomatous type (150×, hematoxylin and eosin stain). Note scattered lymphocytes among tumor cells. There is no fibrous stroma.

91

Case 23

ADVANCED CARCINOMA OF THE NASOPHARYNX

Clinical presentation

A 43 year old Chinese man who had a two month history of severe headaches and nasal blockage, later developed vertigo, unsteady gait, and diplopia. On examination, a right partial oculomotor nerve palsy (abducted eye and partial ptosis) was noted. There were no other cranial nerve signs and no palpable cervical lymph nodes. Nasopharyngoscopy showed a bulky, hemorrhagic tumor, arising posterior to the choana and involving the vault and right lateral wall. A biopsy through the right nasal cavity revealed a squamous cell carcinoma.

Radiologic findings and treatment planning

A CT scan (not shown) demonstrated a large enhancing mass, centered in the right sphenoid sinus, and extending from the nasopharynx up to the parasellar region.

Axial (Figures 23A & B), coronal (Figure 23C), and sagittal (Figures 23D & E) MR images were obtained and showed a nasopharyngeal mass (of intermediate to low SI on the T_1-CW images and of heterogeneous SI, dominated by large areas of high SI, on the T_2-CW images) that bilaterally involved the sphenoid sinus, cavernous sinus, posterior ethmoidal cells, and posterior nasal cavity, and pterygopalatine fossa. These structures were more involved on the right than on the left side. There was destruction of the clivus and sella turcica with superior displacement of the pituitary gland. This tumor was staged as a T4bNOMO squamous cell carcinoma of the nasopharynx and could only be treated by radiotherapy.

Histological findings

A biopsy from the nasopharynx (Figure 23F) showed tumor cells of intermediate size with numerous mitoses arranged in sheets, nests, and strands, with occasional spindle cell areas. The histopathologic findings were consistent with undifferentiated carcinoma, lymphoepitheliomatous type. The stroma of this tumor consisted of areas of fibroblastic proliferation, alternating with areas of myxoid substance, and inflammatory cells. The stroma composed ten to fifteen percent of this very cellular tumor.

Comments

As demonstrated in Case 22, sagittal MRI optimally delineates the lesion in relation to the sella turcica, sphenoid sinus, and clivus, as well as its extension into the remaining nasopharynx and ethmoid air cells. Additionally, intracranial extension into the prepontine cistern is optimally demonstrated.

The anatomy, particularly the cavernous sinus, is better seen on MR than on CT. In this patient, the more extensive involvement of the right cavernous sinus correlated well with the clinical finding of a right third nerve palsy. The T_2-CW images provide helpful information for determining the relationship of the tumor to the carotid arteries (Figure 23B). The heterogeneous signal intensity on T_2-CW images (Figure 23B) most likely reflects the alternance of fibrous and myxoid areas, noted on histology.

This patient was treated with proton beam therapy and conventional X-ray therapy. Proton beams can produce superior dose distributions, compared to X-ray beams. This results in improved local control and reduced morbidity, by sparing normal tissue and neural tissue. Thus, the adjunction of MR to CT was useful in giving a more precise definition of the target volume to be irradiated [44].

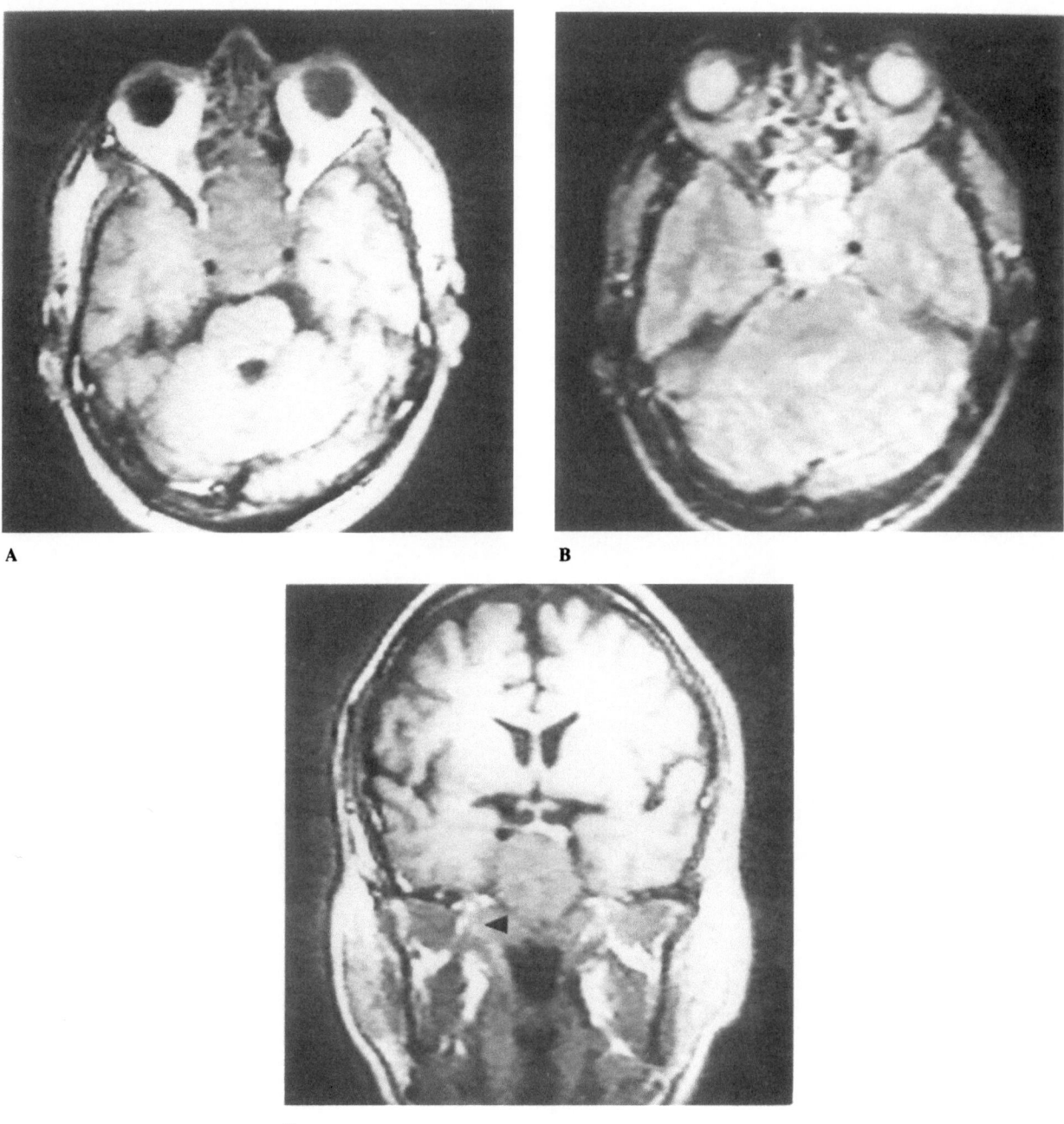

A

B

C

Figures 23.(A & B) *Axial MR projections at the level of the sphenoid sinus* [(23A) *TR* 500/*TE* 20 − NEX = 4; (23B) *TR* 2000/*TE* 96 − NEX = 2. SLT = 0.5 cm]. There is a mass of intermediate SI on the T_1-CW image (Figure 23A) and of heterogeneous, predominantly high SI on the T_2-CW image (Figure 23B). The mass occupies the sphenoid and posterior ethmoid sinuses, invades the inferior aspect of both cavernous sinuses and abuts the carotid arteries. The relationship of the tumor to the carotid arteries is better defined on the T_2-CW images.

(C) *Coronal MR projection through the sphenoid sinus* (*TR* 450/*TE* 20 − NEX = 4; SLT = 0.5 cm). The tumor extends from the nasopharynx to the sella turcica, cavernous sinuses, and mainly right pterygopalatine fossa (arrowhead). Note the normal optic chiasm and pituitary stalk. The most superior portion of the mass is capped by an area of high SI, corresponding to the fatty marrow of the partially destroyed and distorted dorsum sellae and adjacent clivus.

(Figures 23B, C & D are reproduced with permission from [43].)

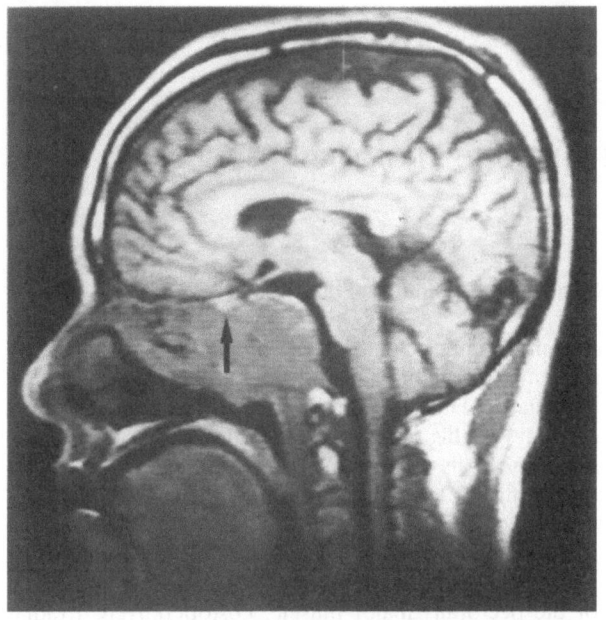

D

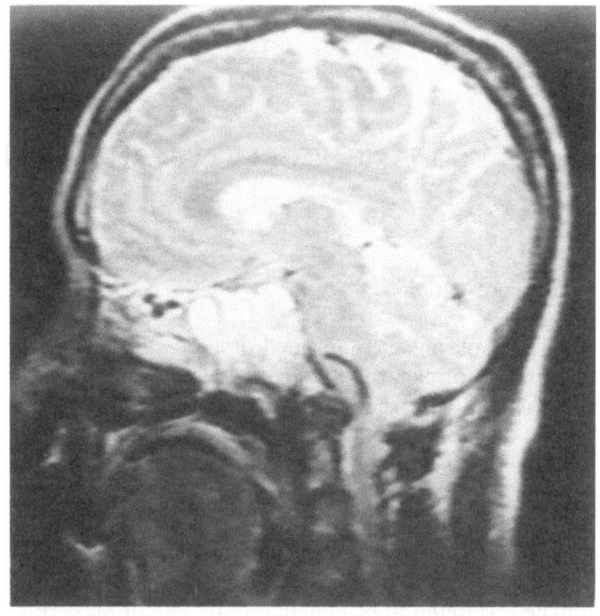

E

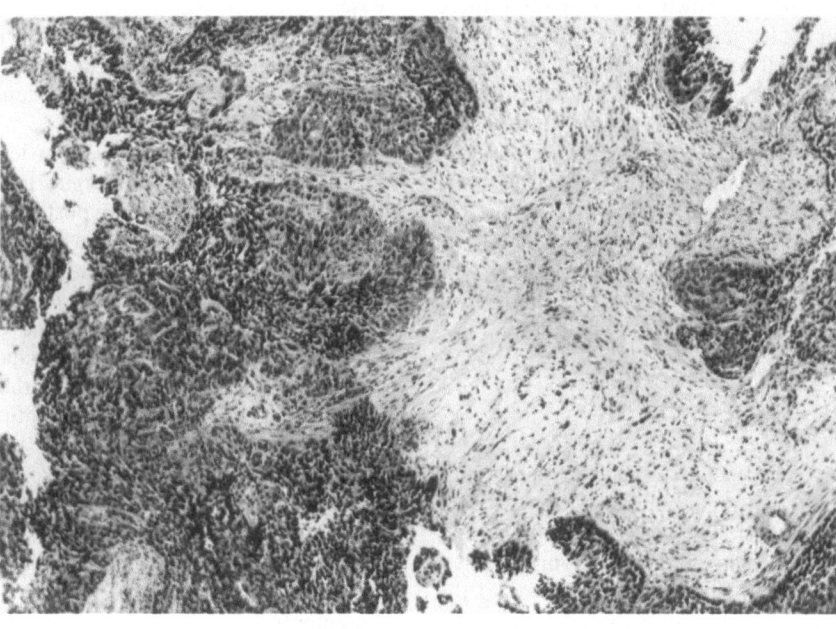

F

Figure 23.(D) *Sagittal MR projection* (*TR* 400/*TE* 20 – NEX = 4; SLT = 0.5 cm) reveals a mass in the nasopharynx, destroying the sphenoid sinus, clivus, and sella turcica, and projecting posteriorly into the prepontine cistern, and anteriorly into the posterior nasal cavity. The pituitary gland is displaced superiorly and anteriorly (arrow).
(E) *Sagittal MR projection* (*TR* 400/*TE* 96 – NEX = 4; flip angle = 45 degrees; SLT = 0.7 cm). This T_2-CW image defines the most anterior extent of the tumor to the nasal cavity better than the T_1-CW image (Figure 23D). This image is acquired in much less time than a conventional SE T_2-CW image (the *TR* is 400 msec instead of 2000 msec). However, the use of a shorter *TR* limits the number of slices that can be obtained. The T_2-contrast weighting of the image is achieved by using a flip angle of 45 degrees and prolonged *TE* [45].
(F) *Photomicrograph of a biopsy from the nasopharynx* shows nests of carcinoma cells and fibrous stroma in this undifferentiated carcinoma of lymphoepitheliomatous type (79×, hematoxylin and eosin stain).

Case 24

SQUAMOUS CELL CARCINOMA OF THE LEFT RETROMOLAR TRIGONE

Clinical presentation

A 64 year old male complained of a left sided oral pain and otalgia for eight weeks. He had a smoking history of more than fifty packs per year, as well as a significant history of alcohol abuse. On examination, there was a very hard, ulcerating tumor mass with the epicenter of the lesion located on the left at the junction with the tongue, the inferior tonsillar fossa, and the retromolar trigone area. There was an ulcer of the soft palate and in the region of the left superior tonsillar fossa. The base of the tongue was found to be adherent to the tumor mass (Figure 24A). The patient had some trismus, indicating pterygoid muscle invasion by the growth. On palpation, there was nodal disease in the left jugulodigastric region.

A biopsy from the left base of tongue, left retromolar trigone, and palate disclosed a poorly differentiated squamous cell carcinoma. On the basis of the clinical and radiologic findings, the patient was staged as T4N1MO. He was admitted for an extended left composite resection, but he developed chest pain and, after cardiac evaluation, surgery was postponed for one month. In the interval, he received two regimens of chemotherapy with improvement, as indicated by better jaw motion and diminished throat pain.

Radiologic findings

A contrast CT study with axial cuts (Figure 24B) showed a large tumor, probably arising in the left retromolar trigone with secondary invasion of the masticator space, oropharyngeal wall, soft palate, paraoropharyngeal space, lateral posterior portion of the tongue, and floor of the mouth. There was a question of invasion of the anterior portion of the left submandibular gland. The hard palate was not involved and there were no lymph nodes in the neck. The mandible was not invaded.

An MR study with axial (Figure 24C), coronal (Figures 24D & E), and sagittal views also showed a left parapharyngeal mass of intermediate to low SI on both T_1- and T_2-CW images, with invasion of the left pterygoid muscle and the soft palate. The marrow of the mandible was not invaded.

Surgical and histological findings

A composite resection (left partial mandibulectomy leaving temporomandibular joint in situ, left partial glossectomy, left palatectomy, and partial left posterior pharyngectomy) of this tumor was performed, along with a left radical neck dissection (RND).

During the operation, repeated frozen sections confirmed remaining tumor near the base of the skull, medial to the internal carotid artery. Plastic reconstruction was performed with a pedicled myocutaneous flap composed of the pectoralis major muscle. Postoperatively, irradiation was to be administered, because of the residual disease.

In the RND, poorly differentiated metastatic squamous cell carcinoma was present in only one of seven left high jugular nodes, with extranodal extension, confirming the clinical staging (N1).

The specimen of the mandible, left soft palate, tongue, and pharynx showed the margins to be free of tumor, but the tumor came close to the posterior resection margin in the areas of the soft palate and pharyngeal wall. There was also tumor at the margin of the gingival buccal sulcus area with diffuse extension into the muscle, tendon, and small nerves. Tumor focally involved the submandibular gland tissue (Figure 24F). The mandibular bone was not invaded, but the tumor extended to the periosteum. Histological sections showed a non-keratinizing squamous cell carcinoma in thin clusters, suggesting an epithelial type pattern, that was associated with extensive fibrosis around the cell clusters. This extensive fibrosis is unusual with squamous cell carcinoma.

Comments

The CT examination demonstrated the soft tissue component of the tumor in great detail, including invasion of the adjacent structures, and the submandibular gland. The mandible revealed no bony invasion. For CT evaluation of the mandible, bone window settings with axial and coronal sections are mandatory.

MRI delineated the superoinferior extension of the mass. The coronal projection clearly demonstrated the lateral pharyngeal wall extension and the medial exten-

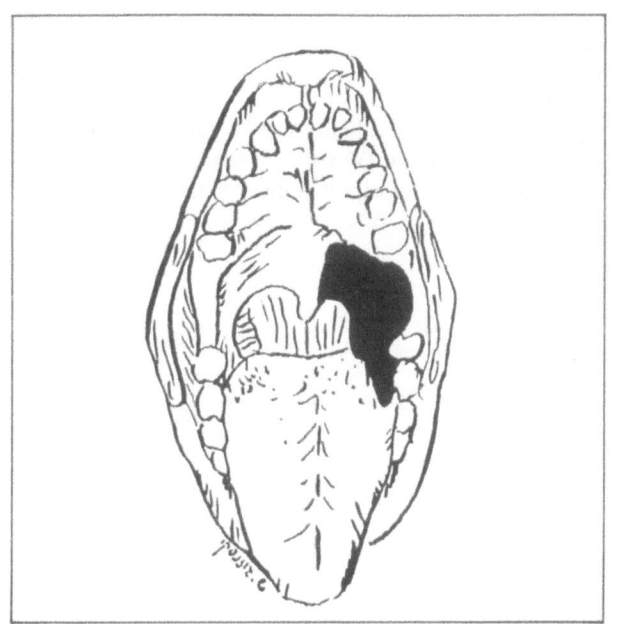

A

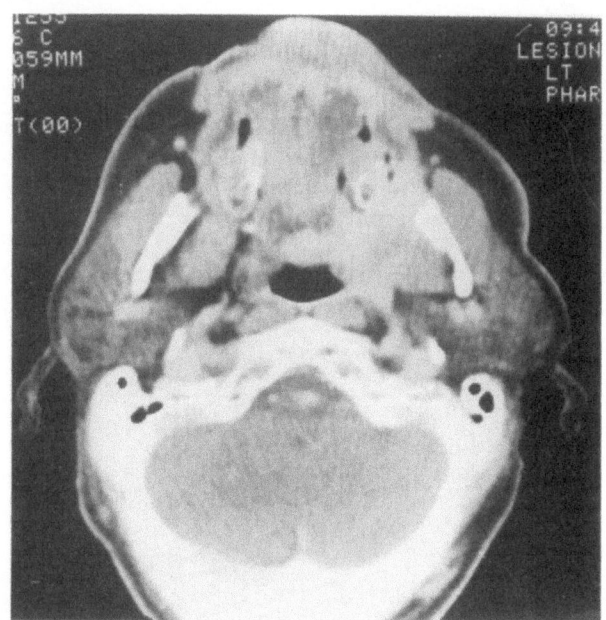

B

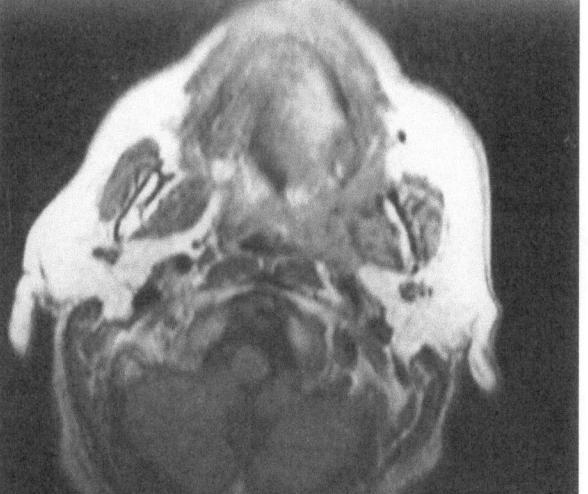

C

Figure 24.(A) *Artist's drawing of tumor extent*, based on the clinical examination with mouth open and protruding tongue.
(B) *Axial contrast CT section through the level of the mid to lower ascending ramus of the mandible* reveals a tumor in the left retromolar trigone with extension into the masticator space, lateral oropharyngeal wall, and left soft palate. There is no bony erosion of the mandible.
(C) *Comparable axial MR image (TR 640/TE 28 − NEX = 6;*

SLT = 0.5 cm) demonstrates a mass of intermediate to low SI in the left retromolar trigone area, with extension to the medial pterygoid muscle and soft palate. The fat plane between the tumor and the pterygoid muscle is obliterated. There are no differences in SI between the tumor and the muscle. The medial cortex of the left mandibular ramus is not distinctly seen, however, the underlying marrow appears normal. This is strong evidence against mandibular invasion.

F. Oropharynx and oral cavity

sion to the soft palate. MR clearly excluded mandibular marrow invasion, but failed to rule out mandibular cortex invasion; higher resolution MR systems might have provided this information.

This squamous cell carcinoma of the retromolar trigone had only low to intermediate SI on T_1- and T_2-CW images, possibly secondary to extensive tumor fibrosis, providing little contrast with the adjacent pharyngeal constrictor muscles, which demonstrated similar signal characteristics.

Marked contrast enhancement of tumors of the oropharynx occur after IV administration of Gadolinium-DTPA [46], and are helpful in the evaluation of the tumor extent.

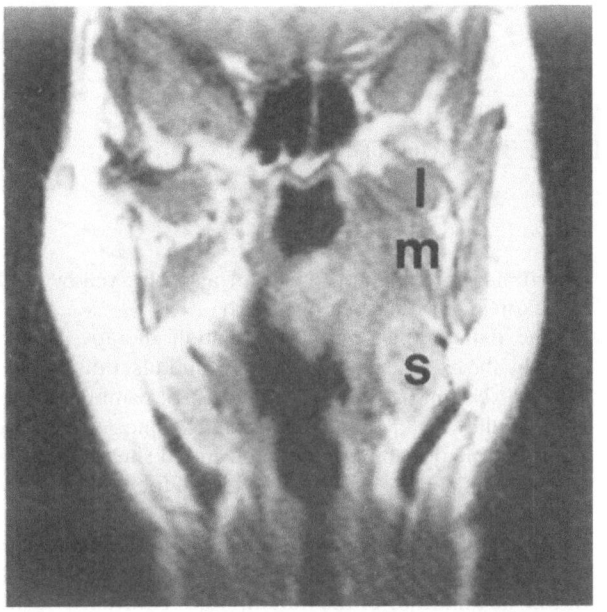

D

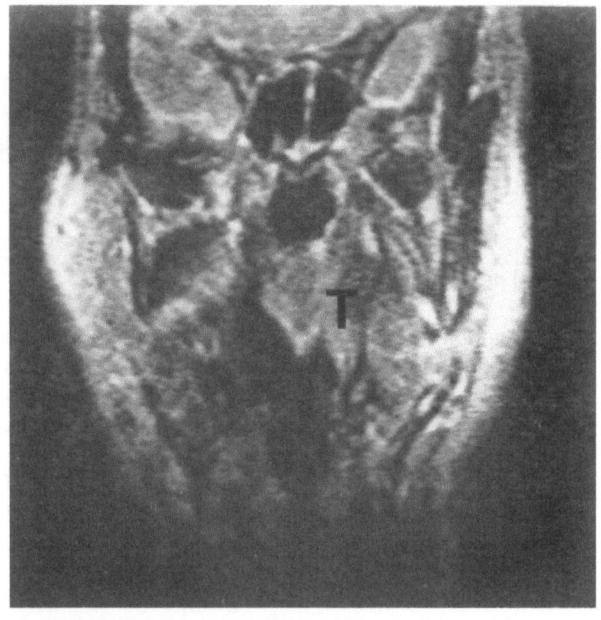

E

F

Figure 24.(D) *Coronal MR projection through the ascending ramus* (T_1-CW) (*TR* 475/*TE* 26 − NEX = 6; SLT = 0.4 cm) demonstrates a left parapharyngeal mass of intermediate SI, extending from the inferior aspect of the lateral pterygoid muscle (l) to the level of the submandibular gland (s), and from the medial pterygoid muscle (m) (which has lost its fatty delineation) to the soft palate and uvula. The mass is situated adjacent to the submandibular gland, superiorly and medially.

(E) *Identical coronal MR projection* (T_2-CW) (*TR* 2000/*TE* 120 − NEX = 2; SLT = 0.4 cm) vaguely demonstrates a left para-

pharyngeal tumor (T) of intermediate to low SI. Image quality is poor due to low signal to noise ratio, which is partly due to the long *TE* (*TE* = 120 msec) that is necessary to generate highly T_2-CW images. Fat/tumor and fat/muscle contrast is better demonstrated on the T_1-CW image (Figure 24D).

(F) *Photomicrograph of a section through the composite resection specimen* (50×, hematoxylin and eosin stain) shows infiltration adjacent to the submandibular gland (upper right hand corner) by small tumor cell nests of squamous cell carcinoma with extensive fibrosis.

Case 25

SQUAMOUS CELL CARCINOMA OF THE RIGHT TONGUE

Clinical presentation

A 64 year old woman, with a history of tobacco (100 packs a year) and alcohol abuse, complained of soreness in the right lateral tongue for several months. She presented with an ulcer on the lateral mucosal surface of the posterior mobile tongue (Figure 25A). There were palpable nodes in her right neck. A biopsy of the right side of the tongue revealed keratinizing, invasive squamous cell carcinoma.

Radiologic findings

The CT study (Figure 25B) failed to demonstrate a tumor in the posterior portion of the right tongue, but revealed an enlarged, necrotic, high right jugular lymph node and a left 3 mm jugular lymph node.

MRI, performed in the axial (Figures 25C & D), coronal (Figures 25E & F), and sagittal projections, showed the same enlarged lymph nodes. On the coronal image, a 1 cm signal abnormality was also visualized at the level of the posterior lateral surface of the right tongue consistent with the lesion seen on clinical examination. It had low SI on T_1-CW images and low to intermediate SI on T_2-CW images. The lesion was distinct from the surrounding tissue and was about 1 cm in diameter.

Surgical and pathological findings

On the basis of the clinical and radiologic findings, an excision of the right tongue lesion with CO_2 laser was performed, along with a right radical neck dissection. The ulcerative lesion of the tongue was 1.5×1.2 cm on the surface, and extended approximately 0.5 cm into the tongue musculature (Figure 25G).

Histological examination showed an anaplastic, invasive squamous cell carcinoma with areas of keratinization and pearl formation, and prominent perineural infiltration. The tumor was very cellular with scant stromal response. There was only one metastatic lymph node in the upper jugular area out of the forty cervical nodes removed. This lymph node measured $3 \times 2 \times 1$ cm, and on

bisection, approximately 1.5 ml of a serous, yellow fluid was expressed from a necrotic cavity.

The patient then received radiation therapy. Subsequently, she experienced severe pain, and ulceration at the tongue excision site was noted. Because of painful and difficult swallowing, a percutaneous endoscopic gastrostomy was performed. A biopsy at the ulcerated site ten months after the initial operation, revealed small foci of squamous cell carcinoma. Because of the recurrent disease a composite resection was done. The right half of the mandible, and the entire right half of the tongue, including the base of tongue and floor of the mouth, were removed. The defect was closed with a right pectoralis major flap.

Comments

Tumors of the tongue are difficult to evaluate because of their unknown depth. In this case, MRI supported the clinical impression of a localized lesion, which resulted in a limited tongue resection. The detection of tongue lesions on MRI is difficult, because of the generally low contrast between tumor and muscle. The SI of the lesion on T_1-CW images, and even sometimes on T_2-CW images, is often low, especially if the tumor has a significant fibrotic component. Tongue motion is often a serious problem affecting MR tongue imaging, as no device is satisfactory for immobilizing the tongue during the several minute duration of most clinical pulse sequences.

For the evaluation of tongue lesions, the following parameters should be utilized: (1) Three MR orthogonal imaging planes, (2) thin slices (3–5 mm, depending on the available S/N ratio), and (3) acquisition of T_2-CW images. In this case, the lesion was only visualized on the coronal images, which are often useful in patients with mobile tongue and floor of mouth pathology. The only positive MR finding in carcinoma of the tongue may be distortion of the fatty planes. Fast scanning methods and the use of a contrast agent (Gadolinium-DTPA) improve lesion detectability and definition [46].

The lymph mode metastases showed intermediate SI on T_1-CW images and high SI on T_2-CW images. The latter finding is a reflection of necrosis within the lymph node, which was confirmed by pathology. The 3 mm left

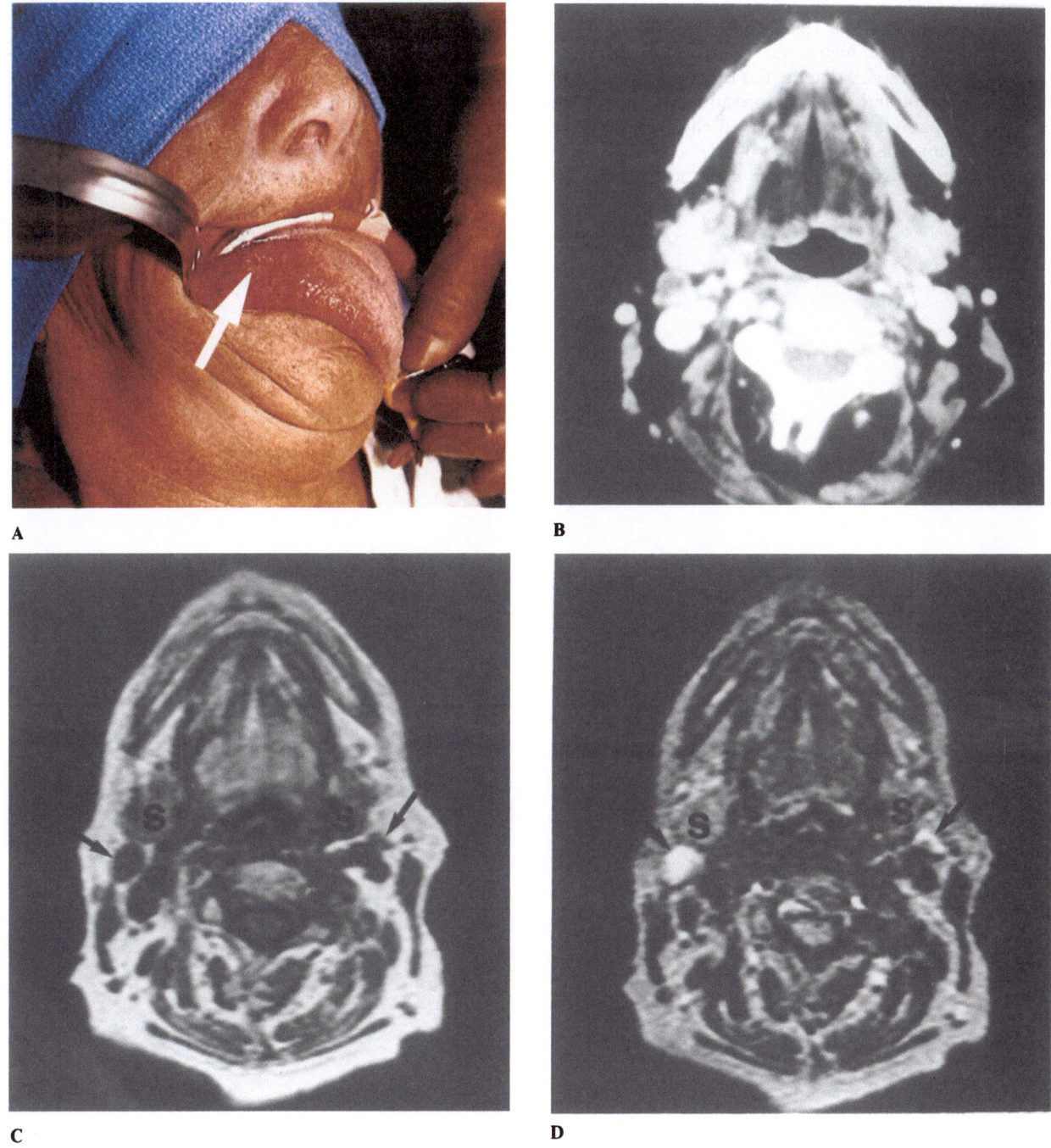

A

B

C

D

Figure 25.(A) *The posterolateral ulceration of the tongue.*
(B) *Axial contrast CT* demonstrates a necrotic lymph node between the right jugular vein and submandibular gland, slightly below the angle of the mandible. The small lymph node on the left side, demonstrated on MR images, cannot be separated from the submandibular gland.
(C & D) *Axial MR projections at the level of the tip of the epiglot-* *tis* [(25C) *TR* 450/*TE* 22 − NEX = 6; (25D) *TR* 2000/*TE* 96 − NEX = 2. SLT = 0.4 cm]. Note an approximately 1–1.5 cm right and 0.3 cm left jugular node (arrows), with rather low SI on the T_1-CW image (Figure 25C) and verhy high SI on the T_2-CW image (Figure 25D), consistent with necrosis on the right, but most likely reactive on the left. Also, note the two submandibular glands (s) of intermediate SI.

F. Oropharynx and oral cavity

lymph node, also had the signal characteristics of an 'active lymph node' (i.e. high SI on T_2-CW images) (Figure 25D). However, by size criteria, this node was not thought to contain tumor and was therefore not biopsied. No left sided adenopathy has been observed clinically in a one year follow-up. The combination of size, as well as signal characteristics, are important criteria in the evaluation of lymph node metastases. High SI on T_2-CW images may be encountered in necrotic metastatic lymph nodes, usually from squamous cell carcinoma, as well as in reactive inflammatory lymph nodes. However, CT aids in the differentiation, in that metastatic lymph nodes reveal a low attenuation center, while reactive nodes are isodense.

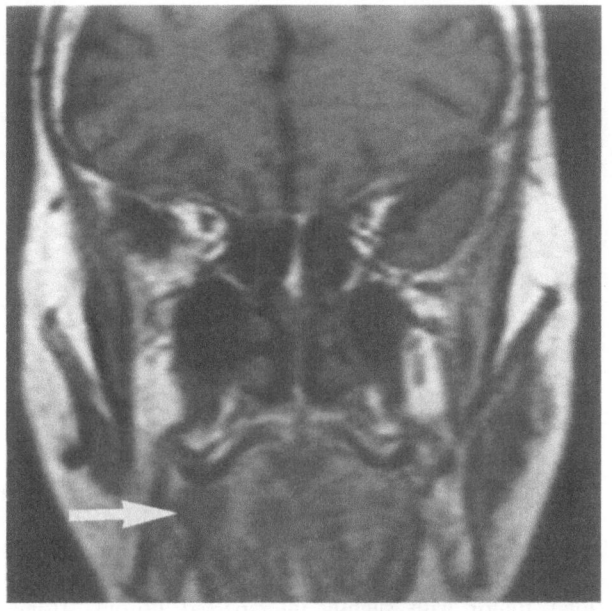

E

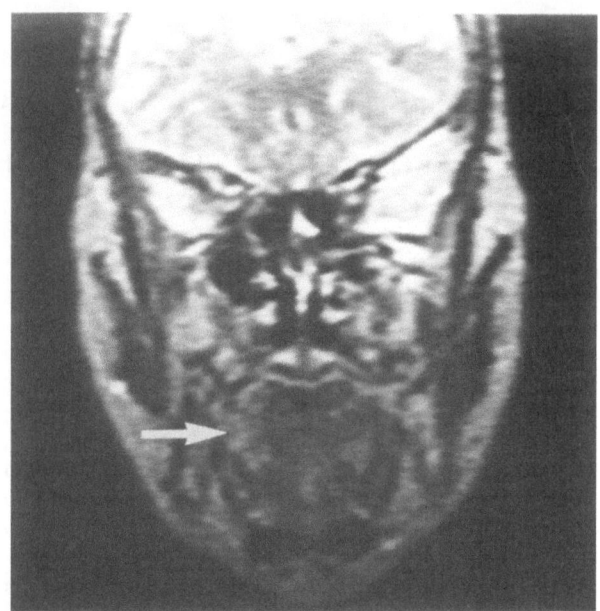

F

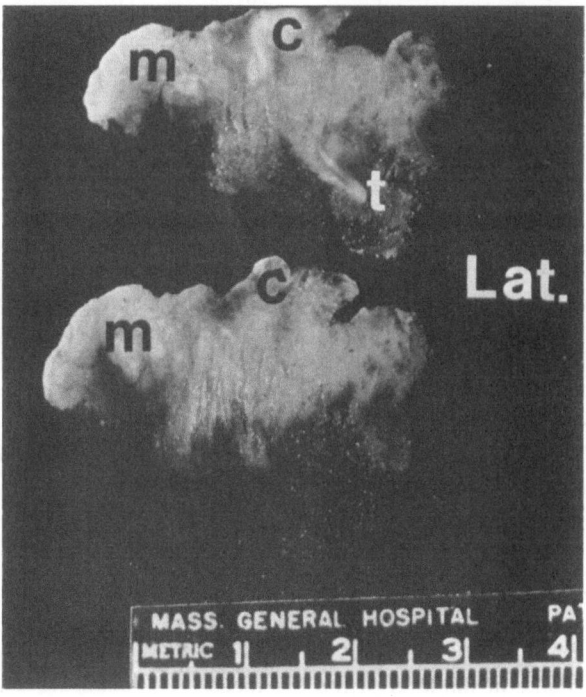

G

Figure 25.(E & F) *Coronal MR projections at the level of the base of the tongue* [(25E) *TR 450/TE 22 − NEX = 6; (25F) TR 2000/TE 96 − NEX = 2. SLT = 0.4 cm*]. There is a 1 cm area of signal abnormality at the level of the right posterolateral surface of the tongue (arrow), that has relatively low SI on the T_1-CW image (Figure 25E) and intermediate SI on the T_2-CW image (Figure 25F). The lesion does not extend to the midline of the tongue and seems to be well delimited within the tongue. There is no evidence of infiltration outside the tongue.
(G) *Photograph of coronal sections of the tongue lesion after excision with* CO_2 *laser* (top section is more posterior than the inferior section). Note cancer (c) adjacent to ulcerated surface area, (m) indicates minor salivary glands, and (t) tendon.

103

Case 26

SQUAMOUS CELL CARCINOMA OF THE BASE OF THE TONGUE

Clinical presentation

A 56 year old male, who admitted to frequent alcohol intake and cigarette consumption, complained of soreness of the left side of his throat for three months and presented with otalgia and dysphagia. On examination, there was a midline mass at the base of the tongue that invaded both valleculae and involved the left pharyngoepiglottic fold. A 1.5 cm right jugulodigastric node, and two slightly smaller nodes in the left jugulodigastric region were palpated. A biopsy from the left vallecula demonstrated an invasive, keratinizing squamous cell carcinoma.

The patient received two cycles of chemotherapy, with near complete regression of tumor in the tongue and resolution of the left neck nodes. There was partial response of the right neck nodes [47]. He subsequently received a full course of radiation therapy to the primary tumor and to the left and right neck. A right radical neck dissection was not done because of a left hilar lung mass which, on needle biopsy, proved to be a large cell carcinoma with features of adenocarcinoma.

Following a left pneumonectomy and removal of positive hilar and tracheobronchial nodes, postoperative mediastinal radiotherapy was delivered. Three months later, the patient had a recurrence of tumor at the left vallecula, aryepiglottic fold, and lateral pharyngeal wall and positive nodal disease in the right upper neck. One year after the initial consultation, he underwent insertion of a gastrostomy tube and received palliative chemotherapy.

Radiologic findings

An axial contrast CT study (Figure 26A) of the tongue revealed a tumor of the right posterior tongue with obliteration of the right vallecular area. There were bilateral necrotic, jugulodigastric lymph nodes at the level of the angle of the mandible that averaged more than 1 cm in diameter.

MRI, with axial (Figures 26B & C), sagittal (Figures 26D & E), and coronal (Figure 26F) views, confirmed the presence of a midline mass at the base of the tongue that invaded the valleculae and distorted the epiglottis, and extended to the left pharyngoepiglottic fold, but spared the pre-epiglottic space. This lesion had intermediate SI on T_1-CW images, and heterogeneous intermediate to high SI on T_2-CW images. Bilateral jugulodigastric cervical lymph nodes revealed intermediate SI on T_1-CW images and high SI on T_2-CW images.

Histological findings

The original biopsy from the tongue base (Figure 26G) showed a keratinizing, squamous cell carcinoma that extended into areas of lymphoid tissue (lingual tonsil) and minor salivary gland structures. It was a moderately cellular tumor with slightly interspersed fibrous stroma. These histological features may explain the high SI on T_2-CW images. However, some contribution of normal lymphoid tissue of the posterior tongue cannot be excluded (normal lymphoid tissue displays high SI).

Comments

CT, in more than fifty percent of cases [48], does not satisfactorily delineate carcinoma within the tongue, especially the posterior third. This finding is probably due to the infiltrative nature of many tongue carcinomas that fail to produce a mass effect within the tongue or a contour bulge at the margin. However, in a small percentage of cases, the tumor is visualized as an irregular, high attenuation mass with or without a contour bulge. The low attenuation midline lingual septum can be utilized to assess midline crossing of a lesion.

Enhancing, occasionally irregular, lymphoid tissue may simulate a tumor, but it is usually in the midline and sharply demarcated from the remaining tongue. Moreover, it is soft on palpation.

MRI delineates infiltrating tongue cancer in a comparatively high percentage of cases [49]. The T_2-CW images best demonstrate the extent of the tumor, by virtue of the increased contrast compared to T_1-CW images. This is especially well seen on the sagittal sections, which are mandatory for tumors of the tongue base (Figures 26D & E). Furthermore, sagittal images depict the tumor contour bulge from the posterior surface, and the extension into the valleculae and pre-epiglottic space. For evaluation of the lateral extent, including midline crossing, the axial images are mandatory.

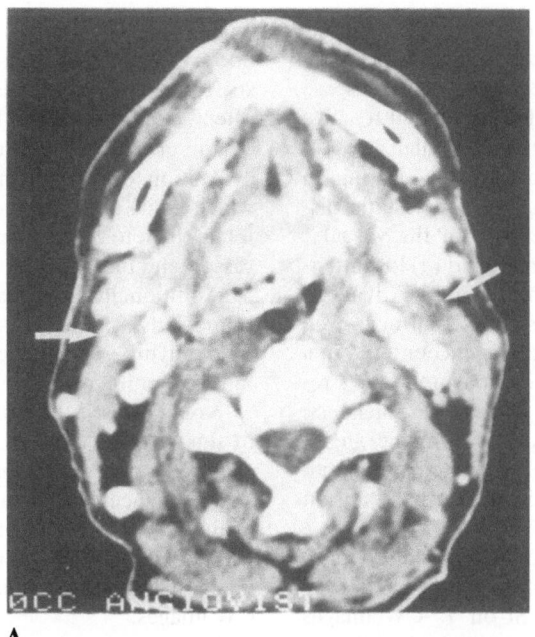

A

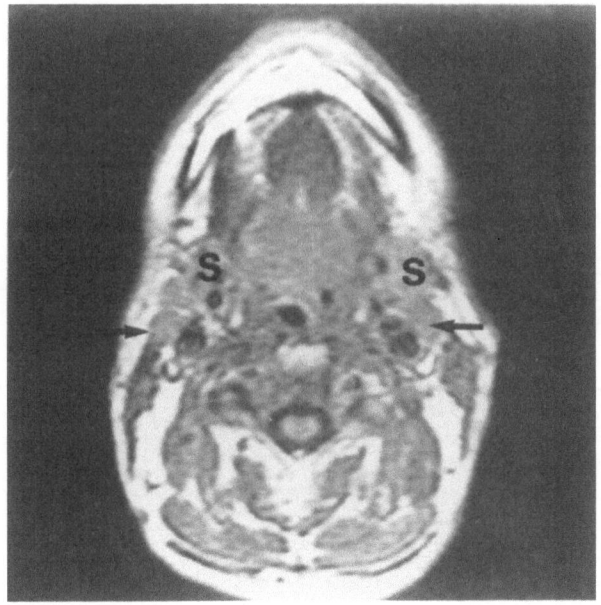

B

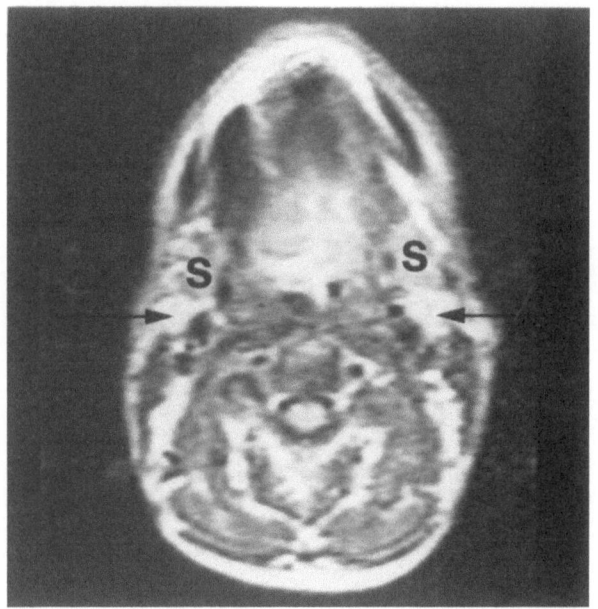

C

Figure 26.(A) *Axial contrast CT section through the base of the tongue* reveals a slightly enhancing mass with extension into the right vallecular area and middle third of the tongue. The lesion obliterates the lingual septum in its mid and posterior portion. There are bilateral necrotic lymph nodes measuring about 1 cm in diameter adjacent to the vascular sheath anteriorly and laterally (arrows).
(B & C) *Axial MR projections at a comparable level* [(26B) *TR* 450/*TE* 22 − NEX = 6; (26C) *TR* 2000/*TE* 48 − NEX = 2. SLT

= 0.5 cm] reveal a mass at the base of the tongue, distorting the epiglottis with bilateral anterior cervical lymph nodes (arrows). The mass and the lymph nodes have intermediate SI and intermediate to high SI, respectively on the T_1-CW image (Figure 26B) and the mildly T_2-CW image (Figure 26C). These nodes are almost indistinguishable from the submandibular glands (s) on the T_1-CW image (Figure 26B), but have a much higher SI on the T_2-CW image (Figure 26C) separating them from the submandibular gland.

F. Oropharynx and oral cavity

In regard to metastatic neck lymph nodes, the following CT criteria apply [50]: (1) size – any lymph node larger than 1.5 cm may be suspected of metastatic disease in a high percentage of cases, with the caveat that reactive lymph nodes, on occasion, may attain a similar size, (2) matted lymph nodes of 0.5 to 1 cm in size covering an aggregate area of 3 cm are suggestive of metastatic disease, (3) obliteration of fat planes and of the vascular sheath in lymph node containing areas, and (4) low attenuation, necrotic areas within lymph nodes. Advanced necrosis of a lymph node with a smooth wall may even simulate a cyst (see Case 35), but this is encountered in a small percentage of cases. Most necrotic lymph nodes reveal an irregular wall with a wall of variable thickness. Large matted, necrotic lymph nodes may mimic an inflammatory abscess; however, the associated inflammatory reaction of the surrounding tissue is usually absent with metastatic lymph nodes.

MR is equally capable of detecting metastatic lymph nodes, that usually have intermediate to low SI on T_1-CW images, and intermediate or high SI on T_2-CW images according to histological composition. Additionally, on T_2-CW images, the interface between the enlarged lymph node and the adjacent neck structures (muscles, vascular structures, submandibular glands – see Figure 23C) is often better depicted on MRI than on CT. Moreover, MRI of the neck allows direct coronal imaging (especially, evaluation of disease in the superoinferior dimension), which helps to locate metastatic lymph nodes and better relate them to the adjacent anatomic structures, especially vessels and the spine.

Additionally, on these coronal images, the size and shape of lymph nodes is better demonstrated. The mapping of lymph nodes often provides the surgeon with useful information prior to radical neck dissection.

Noncontrast MR was superior to CT in the evaluation of this base of tongue carcinoma. Gadolinium-DTPA is especially indicated in tongue and pharyngeal carcinomas, since enhancement of the lesion secures better definition of the tumor [46]. It is anticipated that some carcinomas, with significant interspersed fibrosis, may defy enhancement. Such tumors also fail to demonstrate high SI on T_2-CW images.

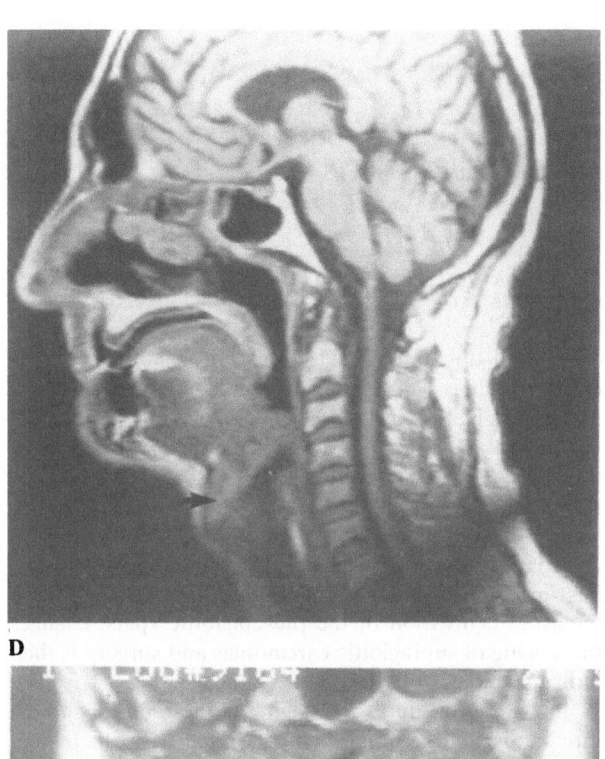

D

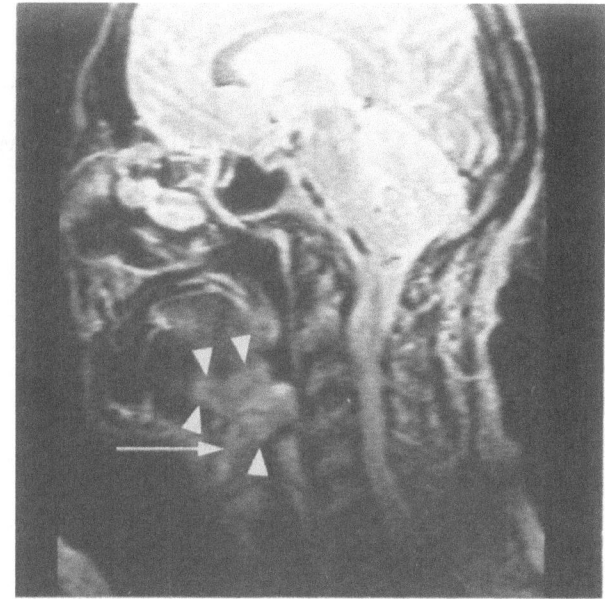

E

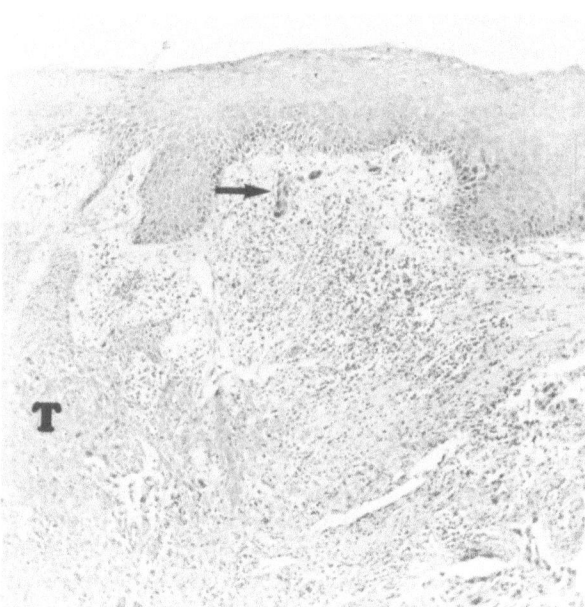

F

G

Figure 26.(D & E) *Sagittal MR projections* [(26D) *TR* 450/*TE* 22 − NEX = 6; (26E) *TR* 2000/*TE* 96, NEX = 2. SLT = 0.4 cm]. A mass of rather low SI on the T_1-CW image (Figure 26D) and of heterogenous intermediate and high SI (arrowheads) on the T_2-CW image (Figure 26E) is demonstrated obliterating the valleculae and displacing the epiglottis posteriorly. The pre-epiglottic space is not optimally visualized on these slightly parasagittal images, but appears to be spared (arrow).

(F) *Coronal MR projection* (*TR* 500/*TE* 22 − NEX = 6; SLT = 0.5 cm) demonstrates bilateral enlarged jugulodigastric lymph nodes (arrows) along the course of the neurovascular bundle. Note the common carotid arteries (c) and the internal jugular veins (j).

(G) *Photomicrograph of the tongue biopsy* (68 ×, hematoxylin and eosin stain) shows normal tongue mucosa with tumor (T) replacing the subepithelial area. There are areas of lymphoid tissue and tumor in lymphatics (arrow).

Case 27

OAT CELL CARCINOMA OF THE EPIGLOTTIS

Clinical presentation

A 65 year old woman, who was a heavy smoker, noted aggravation of her longstanding hoarseness over the last several months. On indirect laryngoscopy, a 1.5–2 cm lesion on the laryngeal surface of the epiglottis was noted. Both vocal cords were normal and mobile. Both sides of the neck were free of adenopathy. Direct laryngoscopy showed that the lesion extended to the petiole of the epiglottis, but did not involve the false cords. This lesion was staged as $T_1 MoNo$. A biopsy and excision of the bulk of the mass were performed. Histopathologic examination revealed an oat cell carcinoma.

Radiologic findings

A plain lateral neck film (Figure 27A) and a CT scan (Figure 27B) prior to biopsy showed a mass in the mid third of the laryngeal surface of the epiglottis, extending towards the right aryepiglottic fold. The pre-epiglottic space was preserved. After biopsy and prior to radiotherapy, an MRI was performed and axial T_1 (Figure 27C) and T_2-CW images, as well as sagittal T_1-CW (Figure 27D) images revealed edema and/or residual tumor at the inferior part of the laryngeal surface of the epiglottis. The right aryepiglottic fold was thickened, and the pre-epiglottic space was free of tumor.

Histological findings

A biopsy from the laryngeal surface of the epiglottis (Figure 27E) showed a tumor consisting of small, rounded, undifferentiated, malignant cells with scant cytoplasm. These cells simulated lymphoblasts in several areas, but were arranged in clusters and nests (lymphomas show individual cells and not clusters). There were lymphatic permeations by tumor. The stroma was very scant. This small cell carcinoma was similar to oat cell carcinoma of the lung.

Comments

Tumors of the supraglottic larynx are usually squamous cell carcinomas. Malignant lymphomas, adenocystic carcinomas originating in the seromucinous glands, and sarcomas of the larynx are rare malignancies. Oat cell carcinoma is extremely rare in this location [51]. The tumor is radiosensitive and high dose radiotherapy is indicated to achieve local and regional control. Chemotherapy is added as an adjuvant measure, since this aggressive lesion has a propensity, not only for regional, but also for distant metastases. Invasion of the pre-epiglottic space changes the staging of supraglottic carcinomas and surgery is then indicated along with the other treatments.

Imaging procedures for staging of these tumors are an integral part of their management. In this case, the patient only received radiotherapy to the tumor and both sides of the neck, since she refused chemotherapy. More than two years after the excisional biopsy, there was no evidence of local recurrence or of regional or distant metastases. A preliminary lateral neck film is useful for surveying laryngeal pathology, especially lesions that occur in the sagittal and parasagittal planes of the larynx.

In this case, direct comparison between CT and MRI is difficult, since the CT was done before, and the MRI after the biopsy and debulking of the tumor. However, this case and the previous case show the advantage of MRI in evaluating the tumor extension to the valleculae, epiglottis, and the pre-epiglottic space. Although these areas are fairly well visualized by CT on axial sections, the sagittal MR images illustrate, to best advantage, structures in the sagittal and parasagittal plane, such as the posterior tongue, vallecular area, epiglottis, and the pre-epiglottic space with its high SI fatty content. Furthermore, the arytenoid cartilages, and the anterior and posterior walls of the subglottic space, including the anterior and posterior commissures are well demonstrated.

The epiglottic lesion, seen on MRI, can represent post-operative edema (the intervention was performed two weeks earlier) and/or residual tumor. Both of these pathologies manifest with the same signal characteristics (low or intermediate SI on T_1-CW images and high SI on T_2-CW images).

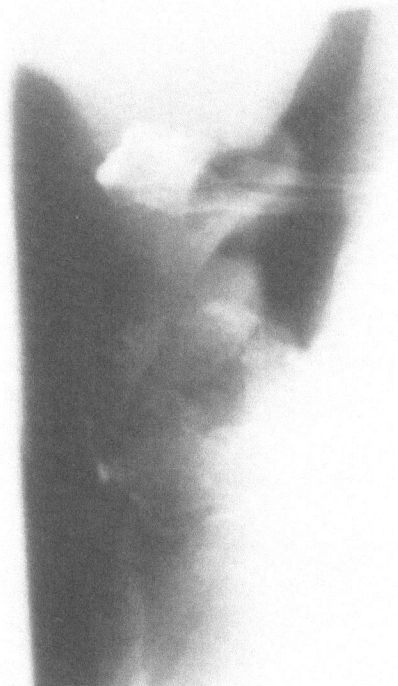

A

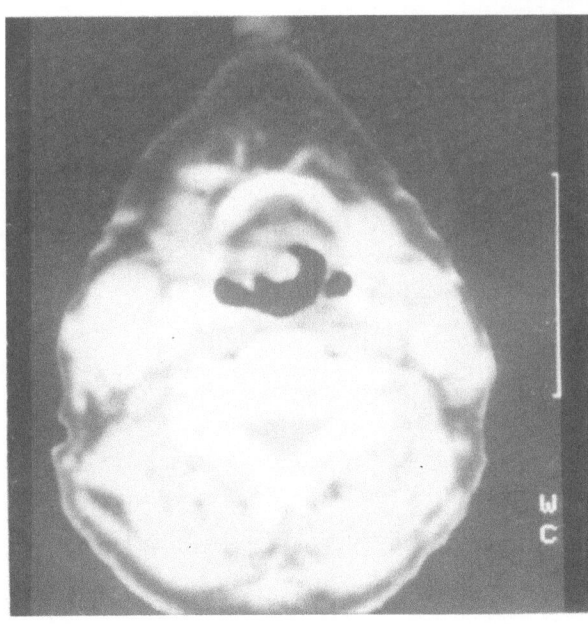

B

C

Figure 27.(A) *Lateral film of the neck, including the larynx (prior to tumor debulking)* shows a polypoid, well defined mass measuring 2 cm in vertical height and arising from the laryngeal surface of the epiglottis in its mid third.
(B) *Axial contrast CT section through the mid third of the epiglottis (prior to tumor debulking)* reveals a polypoid mass arising from the laryngeal surface of the epiglottis, centrally and to the right of the midline with extension to the adjacent right arye-

piglottic fold. There is diffuse thickening of the epiglottis. The pre-epiglottic fat space is normal.
(C) *Axial MR after tumor debulking (TR 500/TE 32 − NEX = 4; SLT = 0.5 cm).* The pre-epiglottic space has a high SI, because of its fatty content and is free of tumor (long arrows). The upper part of the aryepiglottic fold on the right side is slightly thickened (arrow). Note high SI of thyroid cartilage (arrowheads).

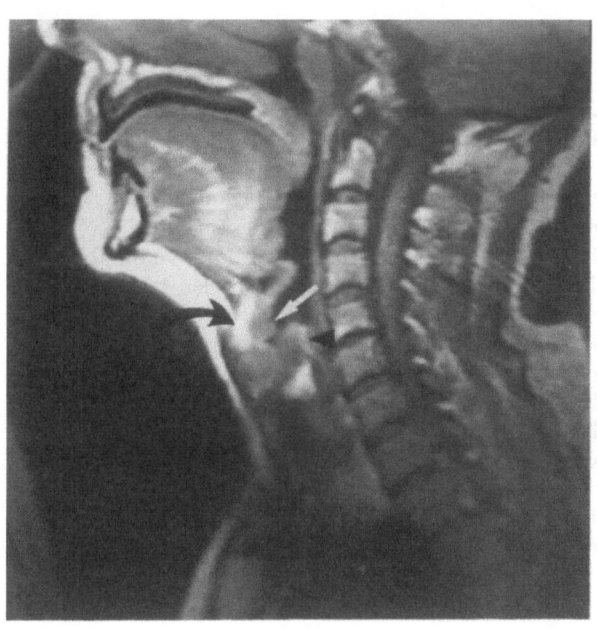

D

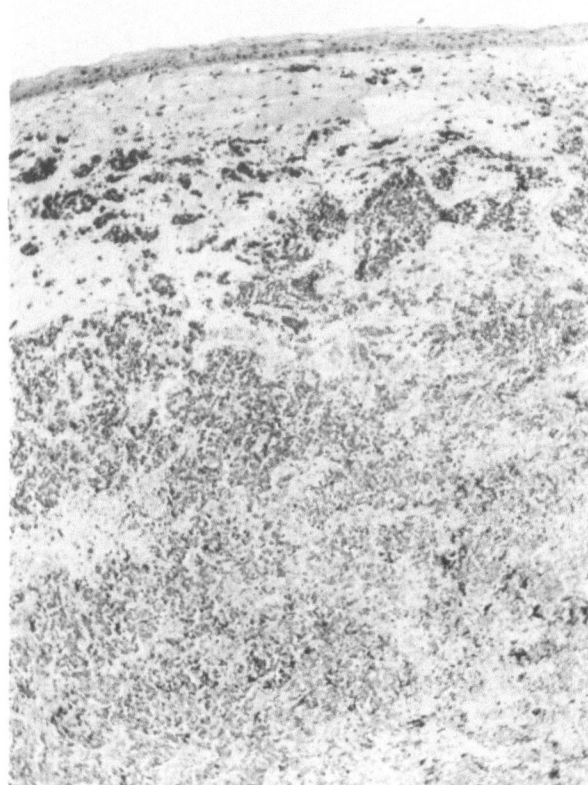

E

Figure 27.(D) *Sagittal MR projection after tumor debulking* (*TR* 500/*TE* 32 − NEX = 4; SLT = 0.5 cm). The epiglottis is shown in its entire length from the valleculae to the petiole. A small mass of intermediate SI (arrow) at the level of the petiole and just above the level of the vocal cords represents postoperative edema and/or residual tumor. The pre-epiglottic space (curved arrow) with its high SI and its classical triangular shape (limited by the epiglottic cartilage posteriorly, by the thyrohyoid membrane anteriorly, and by the hyoepiglottic ligament superiorly) is normal. Also visible is the concave posterior surface of the arytenoid cartilage, which has high SI (arrowhead).

(E) *Photomicrograph of the epiglottic oat cell carcinoma* (80×, hematoxylin and eosin stain) shows the tumor beneath the uninvolved mucosa. Note focal necrosis of the tumor at the bottom.

Case 28

EXTENSIVE SUPRAGLOTTIC SQUAMOUS CELL CARCINOMA

Clinical presentation

A 53 year old man with a history of tobacco and alcohol abuse, presented with stridor after complaining for seven months of hoarseness and dysphagia, with the inability to swallow solid food, and occasional exertional dyspnea. On clinical examination, there was a large, exophytic tumor, involving the left base of the tongue, epiglottis (lingual and laryngeal surface, left more than right), both aryepiglottic folds, medial aspect of the pyriform sinuses, and the false cords. Some movement of the true vocal cords was seen. Mobile lymph nodes, 1–1.5 cm in diameter, could be palpated near the angle of the right mandible and in the left posterior triangle of the neck. The tumor could be palpated under the skin and extended through the left thyroid cartilage and thyrohyoid membrane.

Radiologic findings

Anteroposterior tomograms of the larynx (Figure 28A) and a CT study (Figure 28C) showed a circumferential mass, almost completely obliterating the airway and extending from the base of the tongue to the false cords, and involving the medial aspects of both pyriform sinuses and the pre-epiglottic fat, with preservation of the true vocal cords. Bilateral cervical adenopathy was suspected.

MRI, with coronal (Figure 28B), axial (Figures 28D & E), and sagittal (Figure 28F) views, confirmed the plain film, tomographic, and CT findings, but also showed invasion of the pre-epiglottic space. The tumor mass had intermediate SI on T_1-CW images and very high SI on T_2-CW images. Bilateral enlarged neck lymph nodes were well demonstrated on T_2-CW images, due to their high SI.

Surgical and histopathological findings

Because of impending airway obstruction, the patient was urgently taken to the operating room for a tracheotomy. Prior to the tracheotomy, an endoscopy was performed with biopsies taken from different tumor sites. These specimens showed invasive squamous cell carcinoma. A total laryngectomy, left radical neck dissection, right func-

tional neck dissection, along with an extensive resection of the base of tongue were performed.

Examination of the laryngectomy specimen revealed tumor, diffusely involving the epiglottis with extension into the false cords, pyriform sinuses (mainly the left), and the base of the tongue. Tumor was not found in the anterior commissure and laryngeal ventricles, but completely replaced the false cord on the left. The tumor was composed of squamous epithelial cells with keratinization and marked lymphocytic infiltration in the stroma (Figure 28G). Metastatic squamous cell carcinoma was found in three of the left high and mid jugular lymph nodes. The lymph nodes from the right neck were negative for tumor.

After surgery, the patient was treated with radiation therapy. More than two years after surgery, there was no evidence of disease.

Comments

In advanced laryngeal tumors, the best therapeutic results are obtained with aggressive surgery, postoperative radiotherapy, and adjuvant chemotherapy. Even if there is no suspicion of persistent tumor, chemotherapy seems to prevent or delay recurrences [47].

In large laryngeal carcinomas, imaging evaluation is of the utmost importance for staging, since the surgeon cannot always rely on direct observation through the endoscope.

CT studies of the larynx can only be obtained in the axial plane. Coronal and sagittal reconstructions are derived from 2 mm axial sections, but cannot delineate the anatomy in sufficient detail for accurate evaluation of tumor extent. Furthermore, CT is inadequate for assessing invasion of the vallecular area and of the base of the tongue by supraglottic tumors, because of overlap of adjacent structures.

Likewise, separation of the false cords, laryngeal ventricles and true cords is not possible on CT. Sagittal MR images demonstrate invasion of the tongue, including the vallecular area, pre-epiglottic space, anterior and posterior commissures, and anterior and posterior walls of the subglottic space. Coronal images, either with conventional tomograms or MR, optimally depict the false cords, large ventricles and true cords. Coronal MRI is also valuable

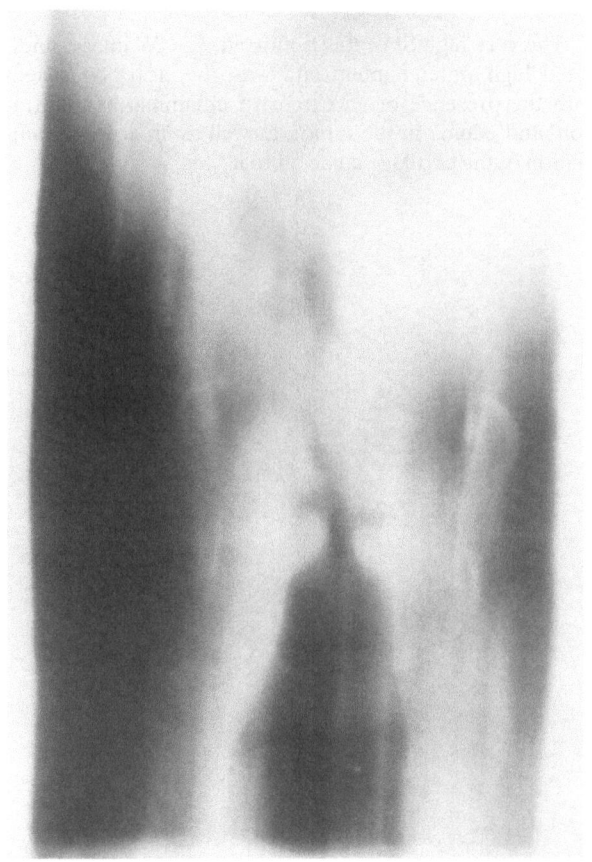

A

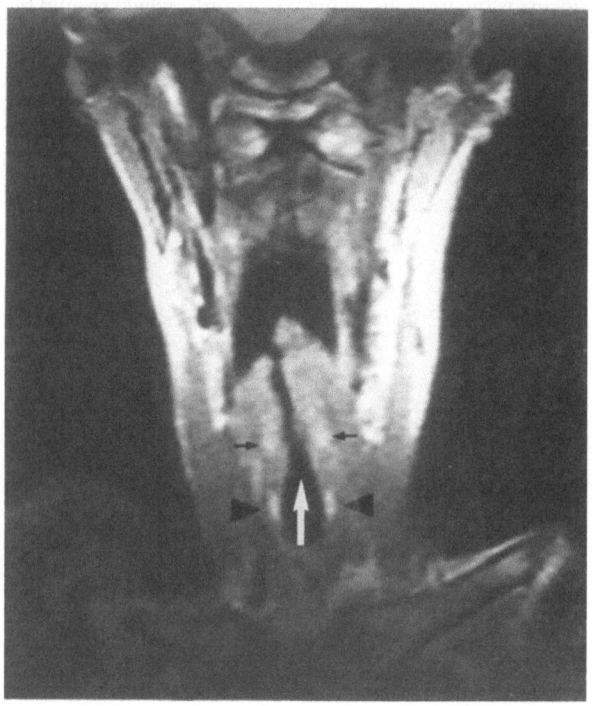

B

Figure 28.(A) *Anteroposterior tomographic section through the mid larynx* reveals a large, polypoid mass which is irregular in contour and involves the epiglottis, aryepiglottic folds, and both false cords. The laryngeal ventricles, true cords, and subglottic space are normal. The tumor bulges into the left and right pyriform sinuses.

(B) *Comparable MR coronal projection (TR 700/TE 21 − NEX = 4; SLT = 0.5 cm).* A large mass of intermediate SI obliterates the supraglottic airway with extension to both pyriform sinuses and the false cords. The false cords (short arrows) usually have distinctly high SI due to the abundance of loose, areolar and glandular tissue [51]. Note normal true cords and subglottic space (arrow), and cricoid cartilage (arrowheads).

G. Larynx

for assessing the pyriform sinuses, paralaryngeal fat planes, cricoid and thyroid cartilages, and the lateral subglottic space.

Another important parameter in staging laryngeal cancers is the mobility of the vocal cords, which should be assessed by conventional fluoroscopy.

The very high SI of this tumor on T_2-CW images indicated high water content and was, therefore, consistent with the presence of an extensive inflammatory infiltration, and edema in the tumor, as well as an acute inflammation of the cartilage adjacent to it.

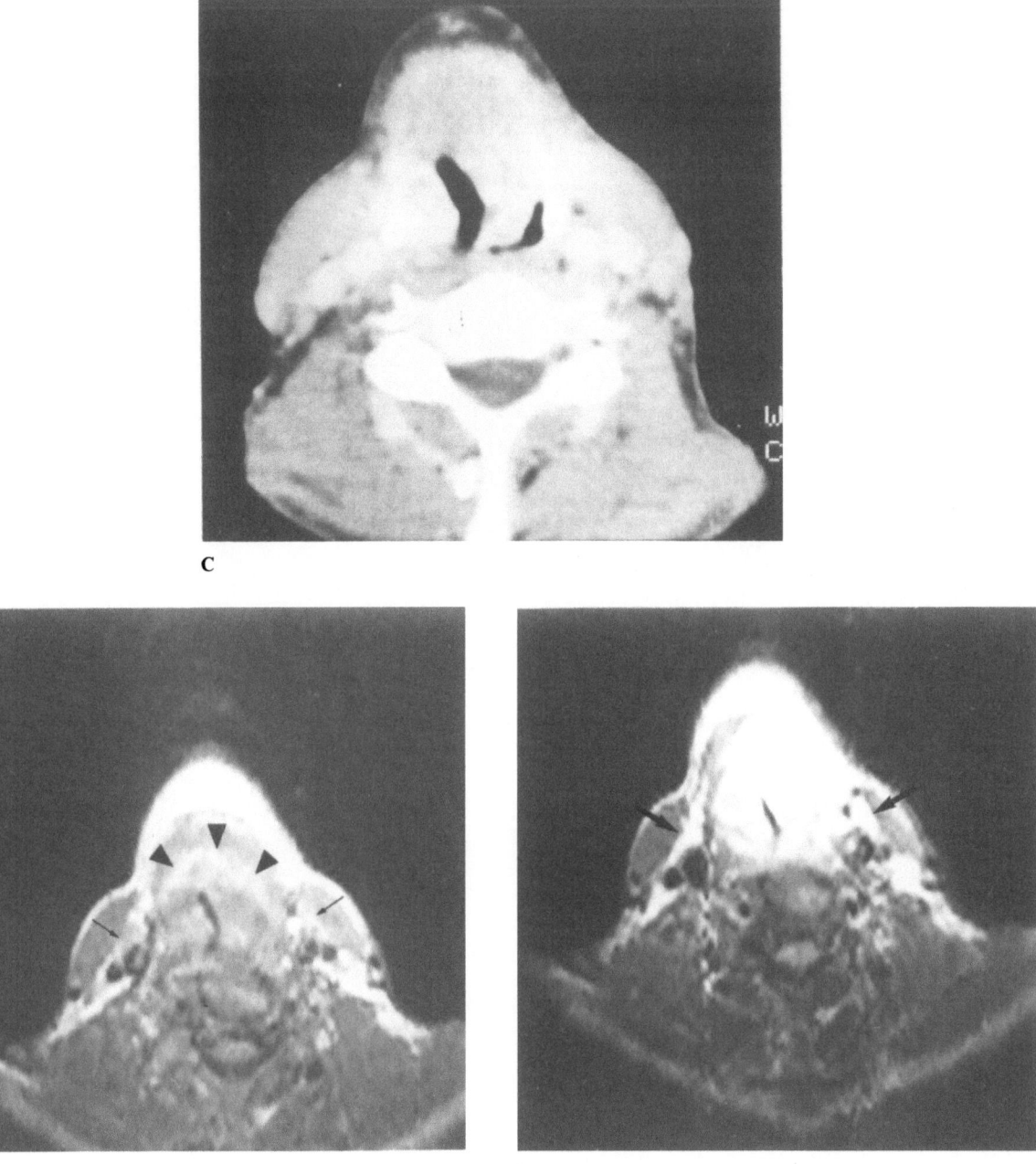

C

D

E

Figure 28.(C) *Axial contrast CT section through the upper part of the supraglottic larynx* reveals a large mass involving the epiglottis and aryepiglottic folds, especially on the left. The lumen of the larynx is narrowed irregularly, and displaced to the right. Note the deformed left pyriform sinus.
(D & E) *Comparable axial MR projections* [(28D): *TR* 600/*TE* 21 − NEX = 4. (28E): *TR* 2000/*TE* 48 − NEX = 2. SLT = 0.5

cm] demonstrate a mass of intermediate SI on the T_1-CW image (Figure 28D) and of high SI on the mildly T_2-CW image (Figure 28E) that almost totally obstructs the supraglottic airway. On the T_1-CW image, the high SI fatty pre-epiglottic space (arrowheads) is obscured by the tumor, which is more bulky on the left side. Note bilateral enlarged lymph nodes lateral to the great vessels (arrows), more evident on the mildly T_2-CW image (Figure 28E).

115

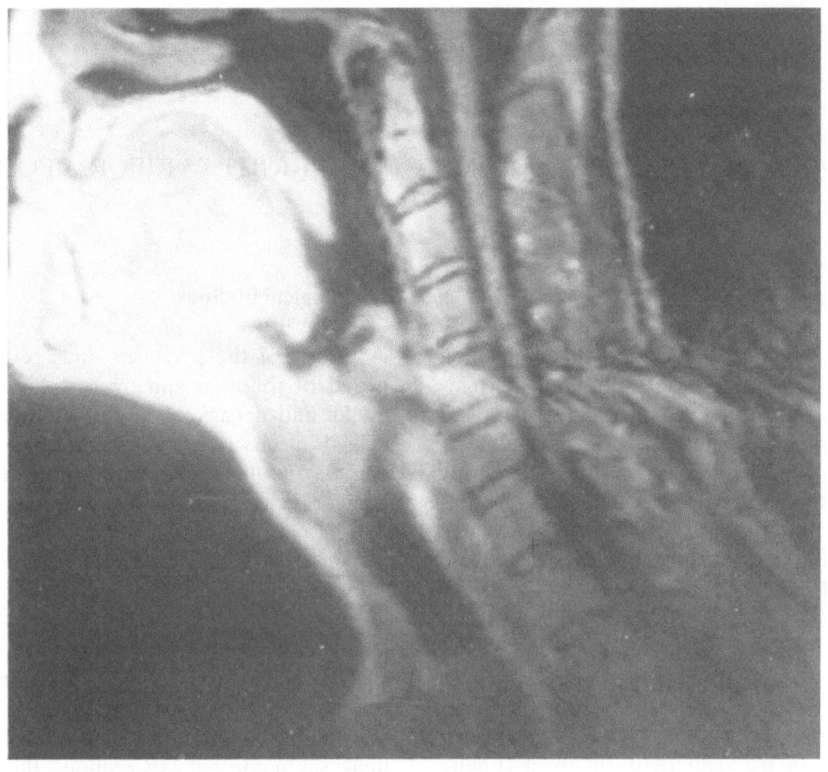

F

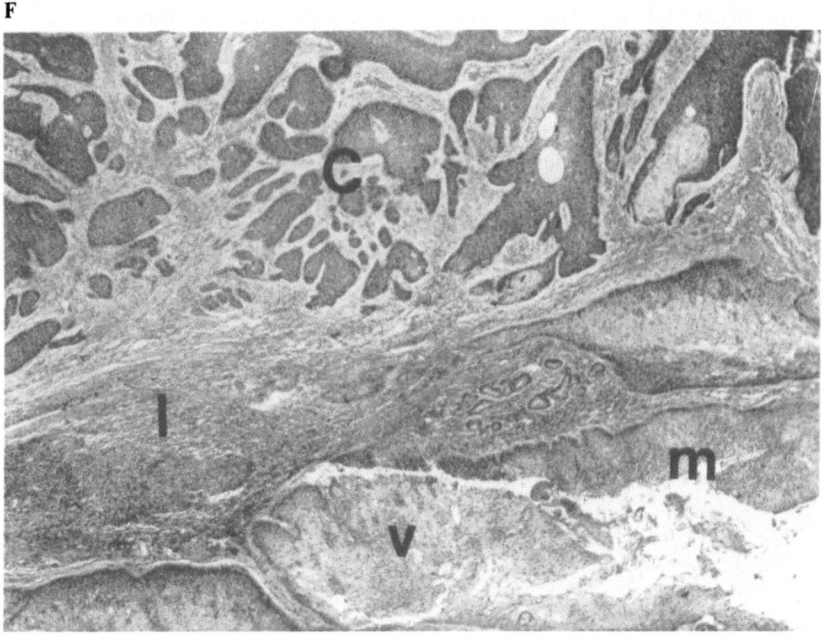

G

Figure 28.(F) *Sagittal MR projection (TR 600/TE 21 – NEX = 4; SLT = 0.5 cm).* There is a large supraglottic mass causing a narrow posterior airway. A motion artifact is seen at the level of the distorted and invaded epiglottis. Tumor invades the preepiglottic fat and the valleculae. A mass projects from the posterior surface of the tongue. The anterior bowing of the tumor indicates destruction of the thyroid cartilage and invasion of the superficial tissues, as evidenced by narrowing of the subcutaneous fat stripe.

(G) *Photomicrograph of a section through the left false cord (50 ×, hematoxylin and eosin stain)* shows invasive squamous cell carcinoma (C), with dense lymphocytic infiltrate (l) in the subepithelial region of the ventricular area (v). Mucosal surface (m).

Case 29

SQUAMOUS CELL CARCINOMA OF THE RIGHT PYRIFORM FOSSA

Clinical presentation

A 56 year old male, who was a heavy smoker, complained of a sore thorat for the last few months. Indirect laryngoscopy revealed a lesion in the right pyriform fossa with normal vocal cord mobility. There were no palpable cervical lymph nodes in the neck. Direct laryngoscopy showed a lesion of the right pyriform fossa and aryepiglottic fold with extension to the false cord. A biopsy revealed squamous cell carcinoma. The patient refused surgery and was treated with radiotherapy.

Radiologic findings

Anteroposterior tomograms, done prior to the biopsy, showed obliteration of the right pyriform fossa (Figure 29D). A CT study of the larynx and neck with axial cuts (Figure 29A) demonstrated an area of increased attenuation in the right pyriform sinus with obliteration of the aryepiglottic fold (AEF). On multiple CT sections, the right false cord and laryngeal ventricle could not be discerned. The vocal cords appeared normal. There were no metastatic lymph nodes in the left and right neck.

MR images confirmed the CT and AP tomographic findings. Axial (Figures 29B & C), coronal (Figure 29E & F), and sagittal views showed a lesion of intermediate SI on T_1-CW images and high SI on T_2-CW images. There was no involvement of the right true cord and ventricle.

Histological findings

A biopsy of the pyriform sinus revealed a tumor composed of rounded and ovoid cells with hyperchromatic nuclei and occasional differentiation towards squamous cells. Portions of the surface mucosa showed in situ carcinoma and ulceration. The tumor was necrotic with focal cellular areas of squamous cell carcinoma.

Comments

In this case, the CT findings only showed increased density in the pyriform fossa. On MRI, the lesion obliterated the paralaryngeal fatty tissue, which is normally high in SI on T_1-CW images and demonstrated high SI on T_2-CW images. On coronal MR sections, this lesion had the definite appearance of a tumor.

Oblique imaging planes in line with the axis of the glottis (angulated axial views, see Figure 42), along with oblique, longitudinal imaging planes in line with the laryngotracheal airway (angulated coronal views, see Figure 42) were used to demonstrate the supraglottic extent of the tumor [53].

The high SI of the lesion on T_2-CW images was consistent with the presence of necrosis in the tumor. The use of high sensitivity surface coils and a small field of view should enable high resolution ($\leqslant 0.5$ mm in plane) imaging of the larynx in two minutes.

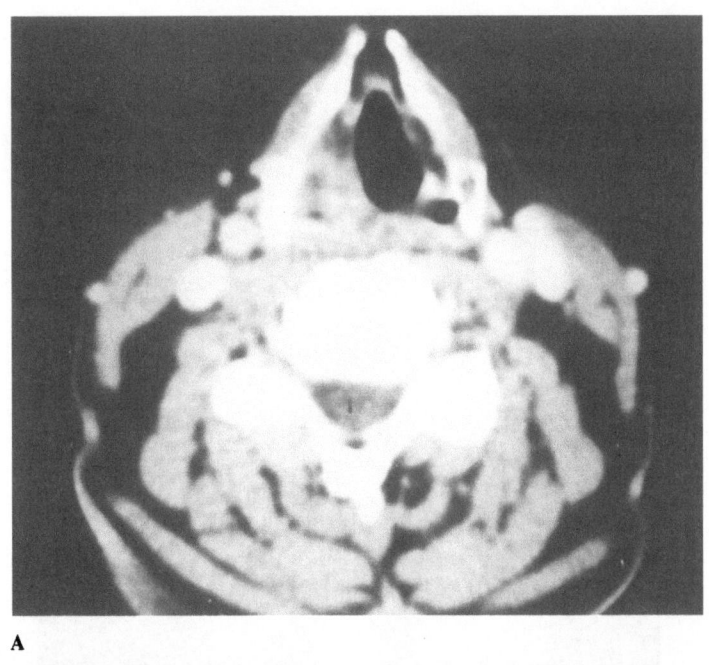

A

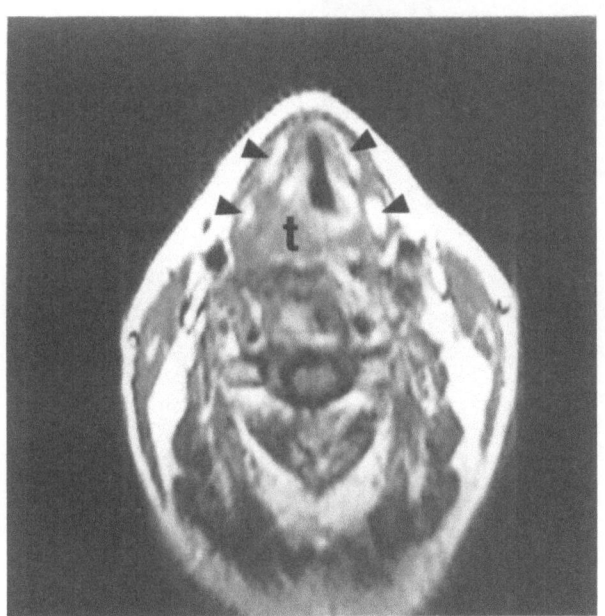

B

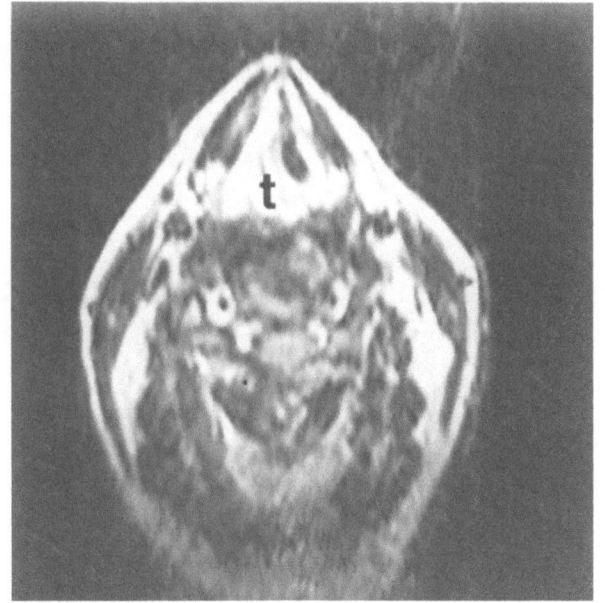

C

Figure 29.(A) *Contrast axial CT section at the mid aryepiglottic fold (AEF)* shows a diffuse increased density of the right pyriform fossa with slight displacement of the AEF medially. The air shadow of the right pyriform sinus is obliterated with the exception of a small pocket in the posterior portion.
(B & C) *Comparable MR axial projections* [(29B) *TR 500/TE* 20 − NEX = 4; (29C) *TR 2000/TE* 96 − NEX = 2. SLT = 0.5 cm]. A tumor mass (t) of intermediate SI on the T_1-CW image (Figure 29B) is demonstrated, centered in the right pyriform fossa, and invading the fat of the right false cord. On the T_2-CW image (Figure 29C), it has a high SI compatible with malignancy. Note the irregular, discontinuous areas of high SI of the thyroid cartilage (Figure 29B) (arrowheads).

119

G. Larynx

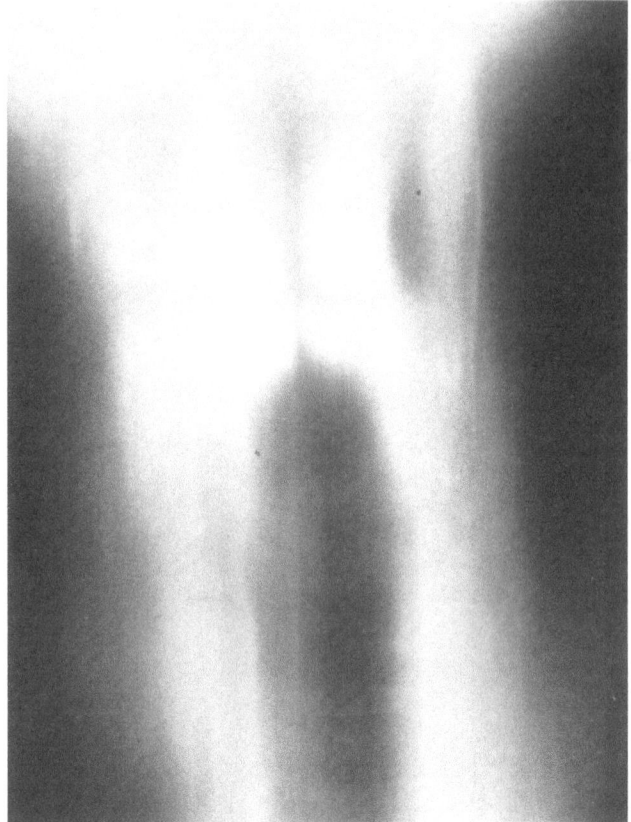

D

Figure 29.(D) *Anteroposterior tomographic study of the larynx in the mid-coronal plane* reveals obliteration of the right AEF and increased density in the pyriform sinus. The right laryngeal ventricle is partially occluded. The right false cord cannot be delineated and appears to be involved by the tumor.

120

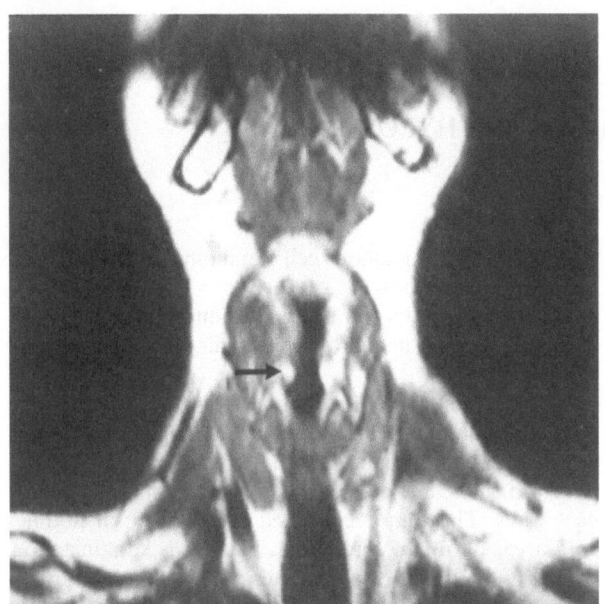

E

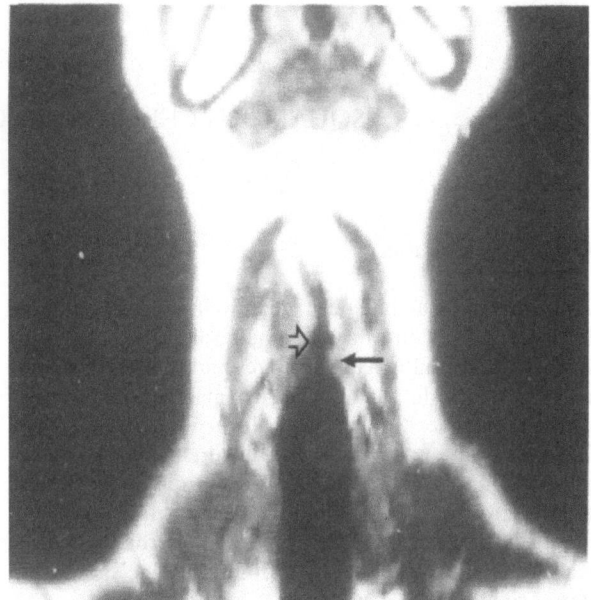

F

Figure 29.(E & F) *Coronal MR projections (TR 500/TE 20 —* NEX = 4; SLT = 0.5 cm) demonstrate the tumor in the right pyriform fossa, invading the paralaryngeal fatty tissue, and extending from the tip of the epiglottis to the level of the arytenoid cartilage (arrow). The laryngotracheal airway is seen in its entire length (except for the inferior portion, which is covered by the posterior pharyngeal wall). This is accomplished by the correct alignment of the imaging plane with the longitudinal axis of the larynx and trachea. Note the demarcation of the true cord (arrow) and ventricle (open arrow) on the more anterior section (Figure 29F).

Case 30

SQUAMOUS CELL CARCINOMA OF THE HYPOPHARYNX

Clinical presentation

A 58 year old man had been doing well for eight years following the excision of a squamous cell carcinoma of the floor of the mouth. He then presented with a well-circumscribed, indurated, ulcerative mass (1.5 cm in its greatest diameter) in the left anterior floor of the mouth. Physical examination revealed bilateral cervical adenopathy. On indirect laryngoscopy, an exophytic lesion extending from the left epiglottis to the left false cord and aryepiglottic fold, pyriform fossa, and lateral pharyngeal wall was found. Biopsies from different sites, showed invasive squamous cell carcinoma.

The patient received two cycles of chemotherapy and then underwent laryngopharyngectomy with a left radical neck dissection. Subsequently, he received postoperative radiation therapy. Two years after this extensive surgery, enlarged lymph nodes with recurrent tumor were found.

Radiologic findings

Prior to chemotherapy, an MRI was performed with coronal (Figure 30A) and axial (Figure 30B) views. The study demonstrated an ulcerative lesion in the left lateral and posterior pharyngeal wall of intermediate SI on both T_1- and T_2-CW images. The lesion extended from the oropharynx to the level of the false cord. A left 1 cm and a right 3 cm jugulodigastric node of intermediate SI on T_1-CW images and high SI on T_2-CW images were demonstrated. The right submandibular gland had intermediate and high SI respectively, on T_1- and T_2-CW images compatible with the increased water content of inflammation, while the left submandibular gland appeared smaller and had rather low SI on both T_1- and T_2-CW images compatible with fibrosis from chronic inflammation or radiation therapy.

A second MR scan (Figure 30C), performed after chemotherapy, showed resolution of the pharyngeal lesion, and a decrease in size of the left cervical lymph nodes without change of SI.

Surgical and histopathological findings

Biopsies from the pharyngeal wall prior to treatment, re-

vealed a cellular squamous cell carcinoma with focal keratinization and fibrosis.

An excisional biopsy from the anterior floor of the mouth contained a microscopic focus of squamous cell carcinoma.

The specimen obtained after laryngopharyngectomy showed squamous cell carcinoma involving the left supraglottic area (with sparing of the left false cord), the left pyriform sinus, and the left lateral and posterior pharyngeal walls. The tumor consisted of submucosal nodules with areas of in-situ carcinoma. There was keratinization, probably the result of chemotherapy. Five high and mid-jugular lymph nodes on the left, removed during radical neck dissection, showed metastatic tumor with extranodal extension.

Both submandibular glands were also excised and revealed chronic sialadenitis with complete atrophy of the acini in the left gland, and acute and chronic sialadenitis in the right gland.

Comments

MR coronal sections optimally displayed the extensive hypopharyngeal tumor. The tumor extent matched the limits of the lesion, as determined from the surgical specimen, histologically with the exception of the false cord which was histologically unaffected by the tumor. MR unequivocally demonstrated the reduction in tumor size following chemotherapy. However, MR failed to detect residual tumor, probably because of the low S/N ratio and poor spatial resolution. These limitations may be overcome with better technologies.

The enlarged, metastatic left lymph node, and the small, presumably reactive right lymph node had high SI on T_2-CW images. Following chemotherapy, the left lymph node slightly decreased in size, while the right node did not change. Moreover, the MR signal characteristics of both lymph nodes remained unchanged. Therefore, as alluded to in previous cases, size appears to be the major predictor of lymph node involvement by tumor.

T_2-CW images clearly characterized the inflamed right submandibular gland as high SI and the left fibrosed, atrophied submandibular gland as low SI.

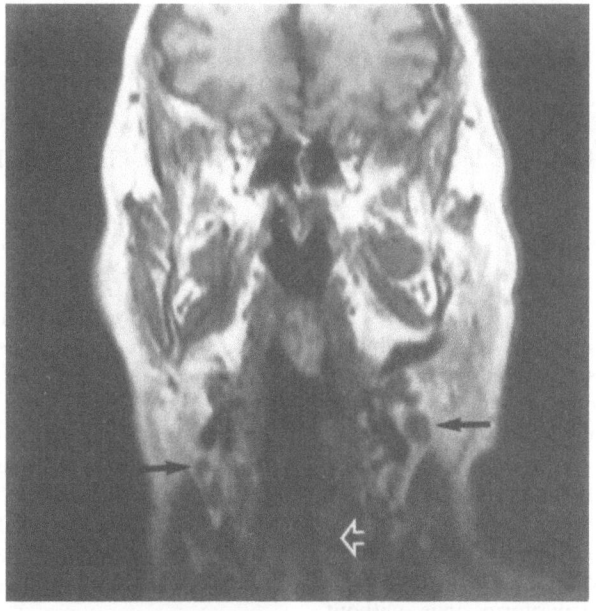

A

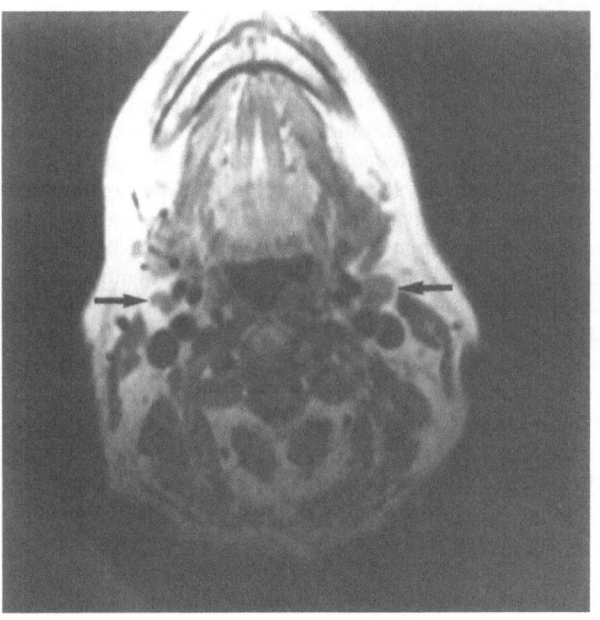

B

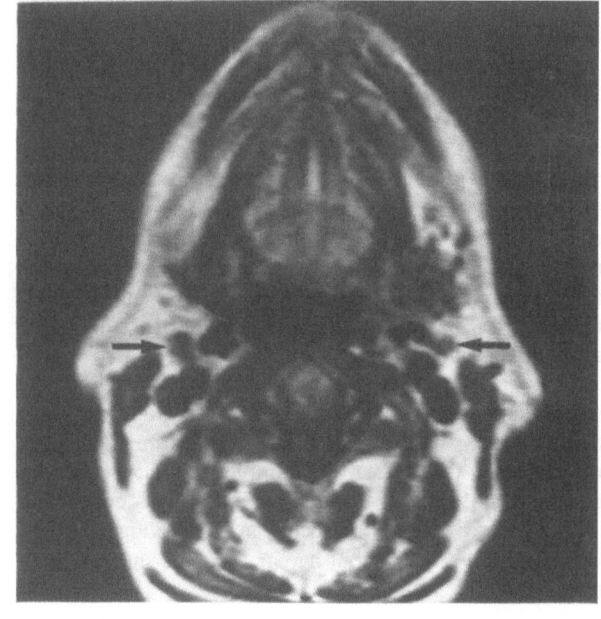

C

Figure 30. (A) *Coronal MR projection prior to chemotherapy* (*TR* 500/*TE* 20 − NEX = 4; SLT = 0.5 cm) displays the pharynx in its full length. The left lateral wall is infiltrated by a mass of intermediate SI, which extends from the oropharynx to the level of the false cord (open arrow). The left pyriform fossa is obliterated. A 1 cm jugulodigastric lymph node (arrow) is seen in the left neck, and a 3 mm jugular lymph node appears at almost the same level in the right neck (arrow).
(B) *Axial MR projection at the level of the tip of the epiglottis prior to chemotherapy* (*TR* 525/*TE* 20 − NEX = 6; SLT = 0.7

cm) reveals a mass infiltrating the posterolateral aspect of the left hypopharynx. The same lymph nodes seen on the coronal view (Figure 30A) are visualized, anterior to the neurovascular bundles (arrows).
(C) *Identical MR axial projection following chemotherapy* (*TR* 400/*TE* 20 − NEX = 4; SLT = 0.7 cm). The left hypopharyngeal mass has disappeared and the left high jugular lymph node (arrow) has slightly decreased in size. The 3 mm right jugular lymph node is unchanged in size (arrow).

Case 31

CARCINOMA OF THE HYPOPHARYNX WITH HUGE RIGHT NECK MASS

Clinical presentation

A 55 year old man, a heavy smoker and alcohol abuser, presented with a two month history of an enlarging mass in his right lower neck, measuring more than 12 cm in diameter. The initial biopsy classified this tumor as a skin malignancy of neurosecretory origin (Merkel cell carcinoma) [54]. A later clinical examination revealed a right hypopharyngeal tumor. On direct laryngoscopy under general anesthesia, the lesion started at the level of the right vallecula and involved the right posterior and right lateral wall of the pharynx and pyriform sinus, without direct invasion of the esophagus. A repeat biopsy revealed an undifferentiated carcinoma. The right vocal cord was fixed.

The patient was treated with three courses of chemotherapy, followed by a full course of radiation therapy, encompassing the primary tumor in the pharynx, both sides of the neck, and the superior mediastinum. Clinically, there was a good response of the primary tumor and the mass in the right neck was reduced to approximately 6 cm in diameter. An examination for metastasis outside the neck, was negative at that time. A direct laryngoscopy was again performed and selected biopsies were taken from the pharynx and pyriform sinus that were found to be negative for malignancy.

The patient underwent arteriography, which demonstrated mild extrinsic compression on the right common carotid artery, without narrowing of the lumen. A right radical neck dissection was completed without carotid resection. Postoperatively, chemotherapy was continued. The patient developed a recurrence overlying his right clavicle and expired about a year after the institution of treatment.

Radiologic findings

The initial pretreatment MRI with coronal (Figure 31A), axial (Figures 31C & D), and sagittal views demonstrated the extent of the metastatic neck mass from the level of the mandible to the supraclavicular fossa, as well as the primary tumor in the hypopharynx. There was no encasement or narrowing of the right common carotid artery. The central area of the neck mass displayed high SI on

both T_1- and T_2-CW images, most likely representing subacute hemorrhage. On the second MRI, which was performed after chemotherapy and at the beginning of radiotherapy (Figures 31B, E, & G), there was a remaining area of abnormal signal in the hypopharynx. The cervical mass had shrunk, but retained the above described SI pattern, although with less high SI areas on the T_1-CW images, and low SI areas on T_2-CW images. These MRI findings correlated well with the axial CT section (Figure 31F) which showed rim enhancement with central low attenuation areas, indicative of necrosis.

Histological findings

Biopsies taken from the pharyngeal wall and pyriform sinus, after the initial course of chemotherapy and radiotherapy, showed chronic inflammation, fibrosis, and edema, but no evidence of malignancy. The excised neck mass revealed displacement of the internal jugular vein anteriorly, with invasion of the wall, but no intraluminal extension. Examination of the fatty tissue in the posterior triangle revealed numerous lymph nodes with metastasis.

Histological examination of the cervical mass (Figure 31H) showed a small cell malignancy in sheets and nests with large areas of necrosis, with peripheral fibrosis and hemosiderin deposits in focal aggregates. Portions of the tumor extended into the skeletal muscle and perineural areas. Final interpretation of the lymph nodes and neck mass was undifferentiated small cell carcinoma.

The differential diagnosis of these small cell malignancies include undifferentiated carcinoma, malignant melanoma, large cell lymphoma, Merkel cell carcinoma, and embryonal cell rhabdomyosarcoma. In this case, the histological features favored the diagnosis of undifferentiated carcinoma over other considerations, because of the lymphatic extensions into the perineural and intermuscular areas, and the absence of melanin.

Comments

In this patient, an operation would have initially included laryngectomy, hypopharyngectomy, and right radical neck dissection. Induction chemotherapy and subsequent ra-

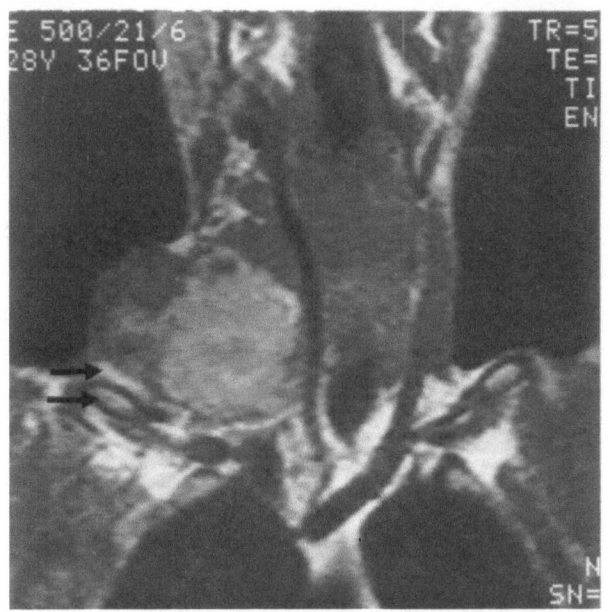

A

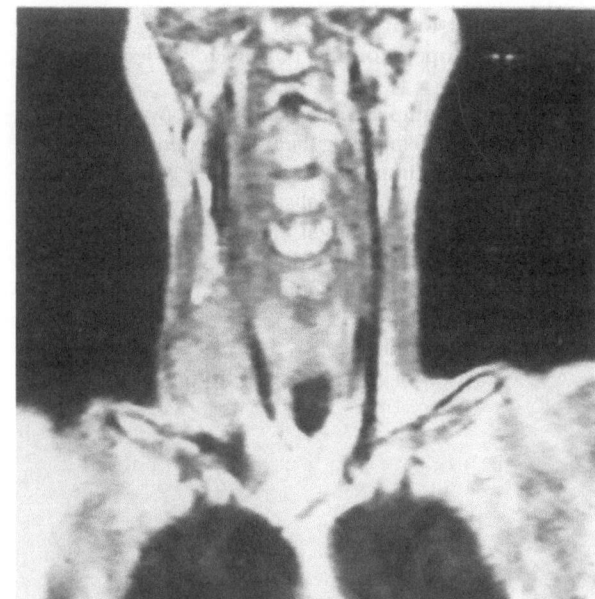

B

Figure 31.(A) *Coronal MR projection at the level of the posterior pharyngeal wall prior to chemotherapy (TR 500/TE 21 − NEX = 6; SLT = 0.5 cm; body coil − the size of the tumor did not allow the use of smaller coils) reveals a large mass in the right neck with high SI of its central portion and intermediate SI of its periphery. The right carotid artery is displaced medially without narrowing of the lumen. The inferior border of the mass is just* cephalad to the clavicle (arrows point to bone marrow in clavicle and to fat in supraclavicular fossa).
(B) *Comparable coronal MR projection after chemotherapy (TR 500/TE 21 − NEX = 6; SLT = 0.5 cm; head coil) demonstrates marked reduction of the mass in the right neck with less deviation of right carotid artery.*

125

H. Hypopharynx

diotherapy led to regression of the primary tumor and therefore, the operation did not include a laryngectomy [47].

Due to its multiplanar capability, MR was more precise, than CT, in delineating the tumor extent. The coronal and sagittal projections demonstrated the longitudinal extent of the mass and a normal supraclavicular fossa. Axial images showed that the right carotid artery was not encased. MR also better outlined the boundaries of the mass in relation to the sternocleidomastoid muscle and the necrotic cavity. Finally, MR helped to monitor the tumor's response to treatment.

A comparison of MR images with the surgical specimen suggests that the areas of high SI on T_1-CW images and low to intermediate SI on T_2-CW images corresponded to hemorrhagic necrosis. The low SI areas on T_2-CW images might be explained by the histological presence of hemosiderin deposits.

The signal intensity of the hypopharyngeal mass on T_2-CW images, after treatment, was generally lower than before, but there were still small areas of intermediate to high SI suggesting residual tumor. As previously noted, however, the biopsy revealed chronic inflammation, edema, and fibrosis, which confirms the difficulty in distinguishing these findings, including post treatment fibrosis from active tumor disease [55–56].

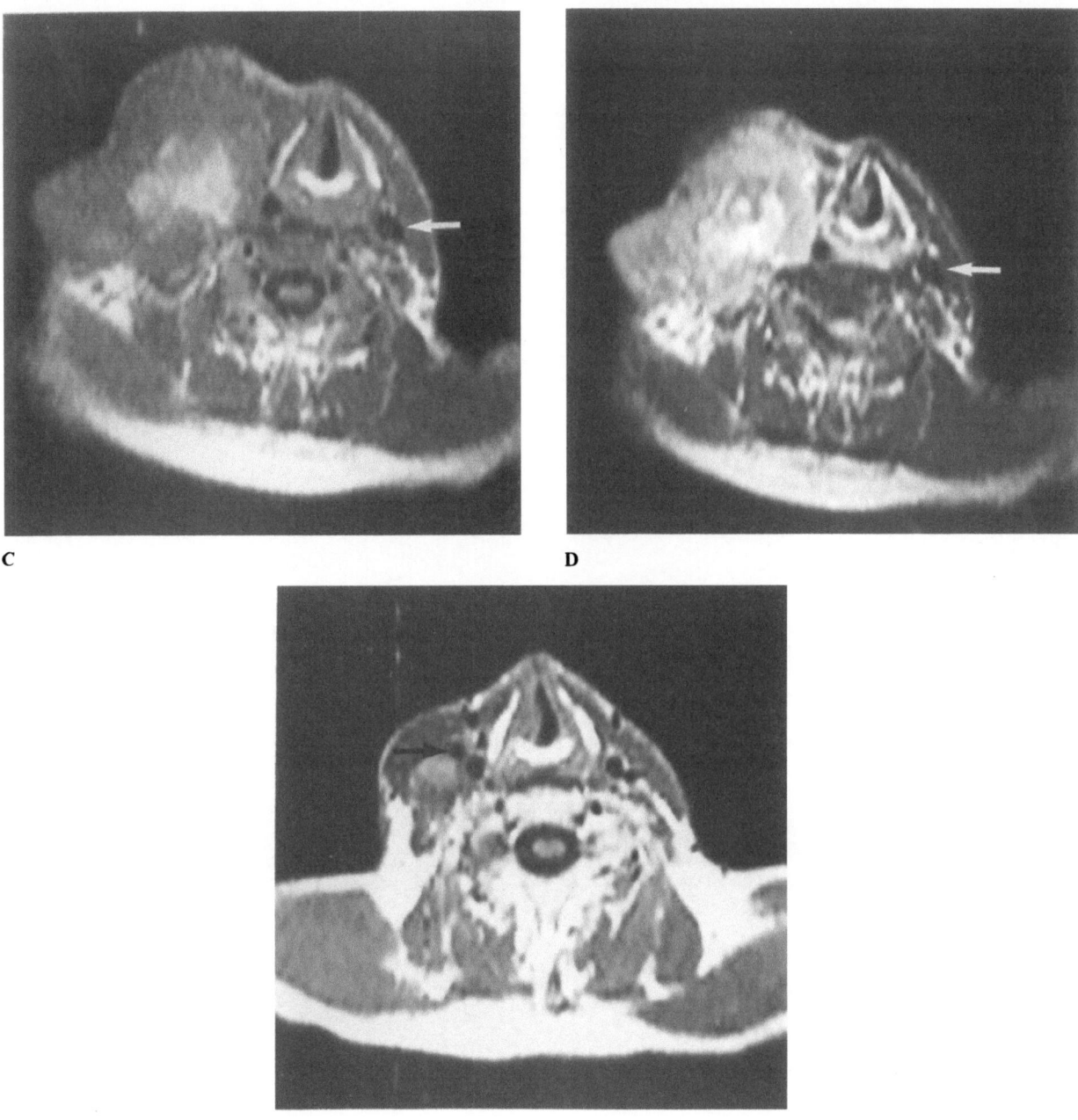

C

D

E

Figure 31.(C & D) *Axial MR projections at the upper level of the cricoid cartilage, prior to chemotherapy* [(31C): *TR* 500/*TE* 21 − NEX = 4. (31D): *TR* 2000/*TE* 48 − NEX = 4. SLT = 0.7 cm; body coil]. A large mass is seen in the right neck with a central area of inhomogeneous, intermediate to high SI and a peripheral area of intermediate to low SI on T_1-CW image (Figure 31C). On the moderately T_2-CW image (Figure 31D), the central part of the mass has some low SI areas; however, it still has higher SI than the periphery. This pattern was confirmed by more heavily T_2-weighted images (not shown). The right common carotid artery is displaced medially, and uninvaded by the tumor mass; the entire larynx is displaced to the left. The right internal jugular vein is not visualized (compare with the signal voids of the corresponding carotid artery and the jugular vein on the left) (arrow). There is a mass of intermediate SI on the T_1-CW image and of high SI on the mildly T_2-CW image which involves the right pyriform sinus, aryepiglottic fold, and false and true cords.
(E) *Axial MR projection at the same level after chemotherapy* (*TR* 500/*TE* 21 − NEX = 6; SLT = 0.5 cm; head coil). There is marked reduction in the size of the right neck mass, which still has fairly high SI centrally. The vascular structure located anterior and lateral to the common carotid artery is probably the internal jugular vein displaced by the mass (arrow). The right vocal cord is in a paramedian position.

127

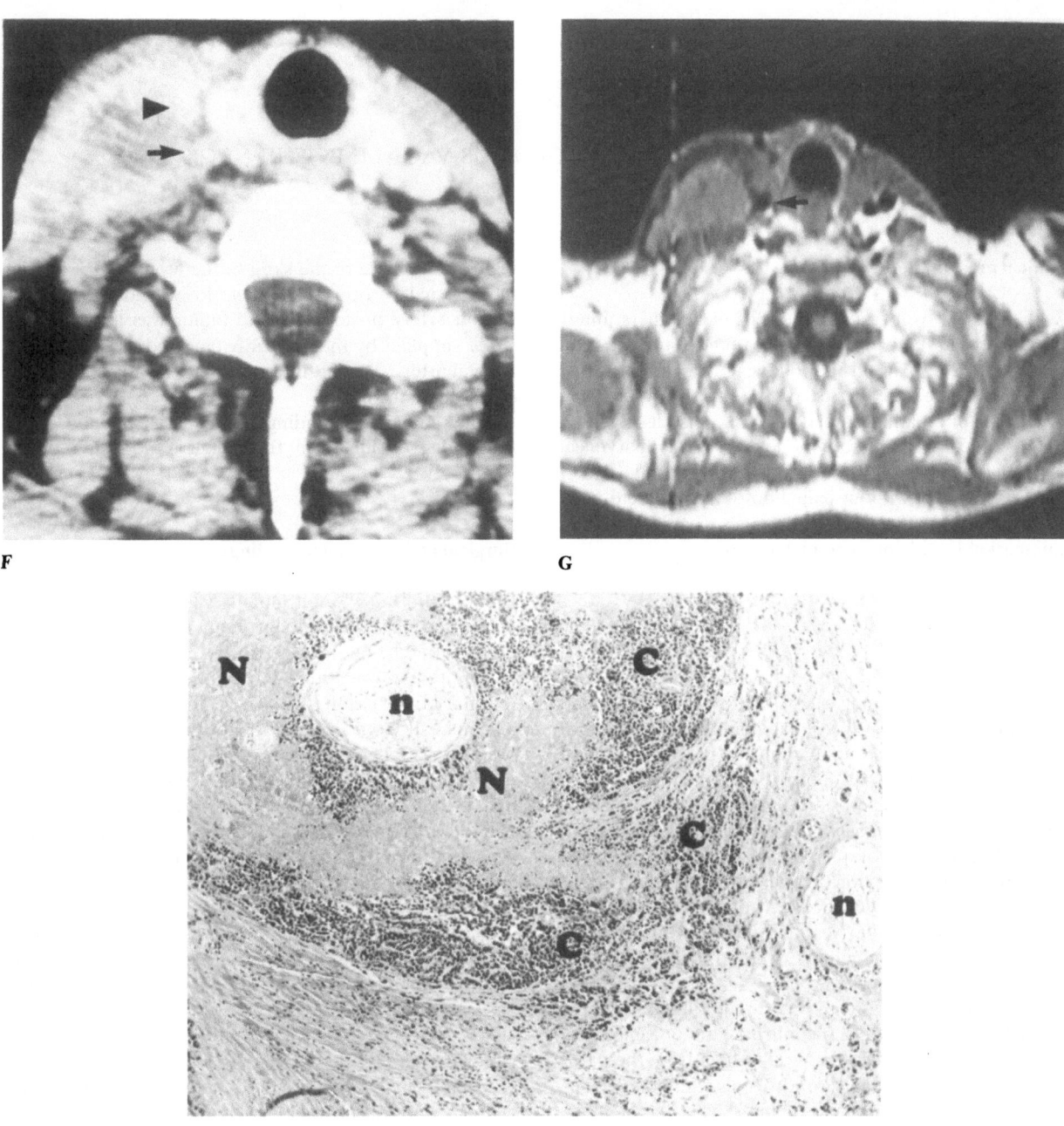

F

G

H

Figure 31. (F) *Axial contrast CT section through the lower neck at the level of the thyroid gland after chemotherapy* shows a necrotic mass in the right neck, invading the sternocleidomastoid muscle. The mass measures about 5 cm in its greatest diameter. The common carotid artery is seen medially (arrow), but the internal jugular vein is difficult to identify (arrowhead), indicating displacement and/or compression.
(G) *Comparable axial MR projection, after chemotherapy* (same machine parameters as in Figure 31E). The common carotid

artery (arrow) is better visualized than on CT and does not seem to be invaded by the tumor mass. The boundaries of the tumor are also better defined in relation to the sternocleidomastoid muscle.
(H) *Photomicrograph of a section through the surgical neck specimen* (72×, hematoxylin and eosin stain) shows cellular, undifferentiated carcinoma (C) with extensive necrosis (N). Note tumor in perineural areas; nerve (n).

Case 32

PARAGANGLIOMA OF THE GLOMUS VAGALE IN THE NECK

Clinical presentation

A 45 year old woman developed lightheadedness, intermittent vertigo, blurred vision, and tinnitus, after several months of neck pain. In the following two months, only some lightheadedness persisted. She had no difficulty in swallowing or breathing, and no fainting episodes.

On clinical examination, the left posterior pharyngeal wall bulged anteriorly. There was fullness in the left anterior cervical area without palpation of any discrete mass or lymphadenopathy. The neurologic examination was unremarkable with intact cranial nerves.

Radiologic findings

A CT study, with axial sections (Figure 32A) showed a large, oval shaped, homogeneous, sharply defined mass in the left parapharyngeal space, extending from the base of the skull to the mid ascending ramus of the mandible and mid soft palate. The mass approximated the jugular fossa, but there was no bone erosion. The lesion could be easily separated from the adjacent deep portion of the parotid gland. The left lateral pharyngeal wall was displaced medially. A bolus injection demonstrated enhancement of this mass along with enhancement of the adjacent muscles. The internal jugular vein and internal carotid artery were not visible on the left and were probably displaced and compressed.

MRI, with axial (Figure 32B & C) and slightly obliqued coronal views (Figure 32D) confirmed the presence of a left parapharyngeal mass that was distinct from the parotid gland and splayed the carotid vessels with no evidence of invasion of the adjacent structures. The SI was intermediate on T_1-CW images and high on T_2-CW images. There were punctuated areas of signal void, suggesting the presence of vessels within the tumor.

A digital subtraction intravenous angiogram (Figure 32E) demonstrated a hypervascular mass beginning just above the level of the carotid bifurcation and extending to the level of the base of the skull. These findings were consistent with a paraganglioma (glomus tumor).

Selective angiography of the left internal carotid, left external carotid, and left ascending pharyngeal arteries confirmed the presence of a hypervascular mass extending from the base of the skull to the level of C-3, bowing the internal carotid artery anteriorly, and the external carotid artery posteriorly. The tumor was almost exclusively supplied by the markedly enlarged ascending pharyngeal artery. The left internal jugular vein was occluded at the site of the tumor.

The radiographic findings were consistent with a paraganglioma, arising from the ganglion nodosum of the vagus nerve.

Surgical and histological findings

Embolization of the left glomus vagale tumor was done with polyvinyl alcohol foam. Four days later, a subtotal excision of the tumor was performed.

The tumor was found to be intimately related to the internal carotid artery. The left vagus nerve was displaced near its exit from the base of the skull, necessitating its excision. The hypoglossal nerve was also compressed by the lesion. In order to achieve subtotal removal, a mandibular split was carried out, which was subsequently repaired with a metal plate. The adjacent internal jugular vein was thrombosed. Residual disease was left behind, particularly at the entry point of the carotid artery to the intracranial space. Radiation therapy to the base of the skull was initiated for treatment of the residual disease.

A cut section through the excised tumor (Figure 32F) showed replacement of tissues by vascular spaces with nests and clusters of small, rounded cells that had moderate cytoplasm content. The cells focally herniated into the vascular spaces. Embolic material occluded many of the vascular channels with areas of hemorrhagic and ischemic necrosis. The peripheral areas of the tumor showed fibrosis and prominent vascular channels. This moderately cellular tumor had pseudoencapsulated portions. All of these histological features were consistent with a paraganglioma.

Comments

CT demonstrates a well demarcated, enhancing tumor in the parapharyngeal space that was easily separated from the adjacent deep portion of the parotid gland. Contrast

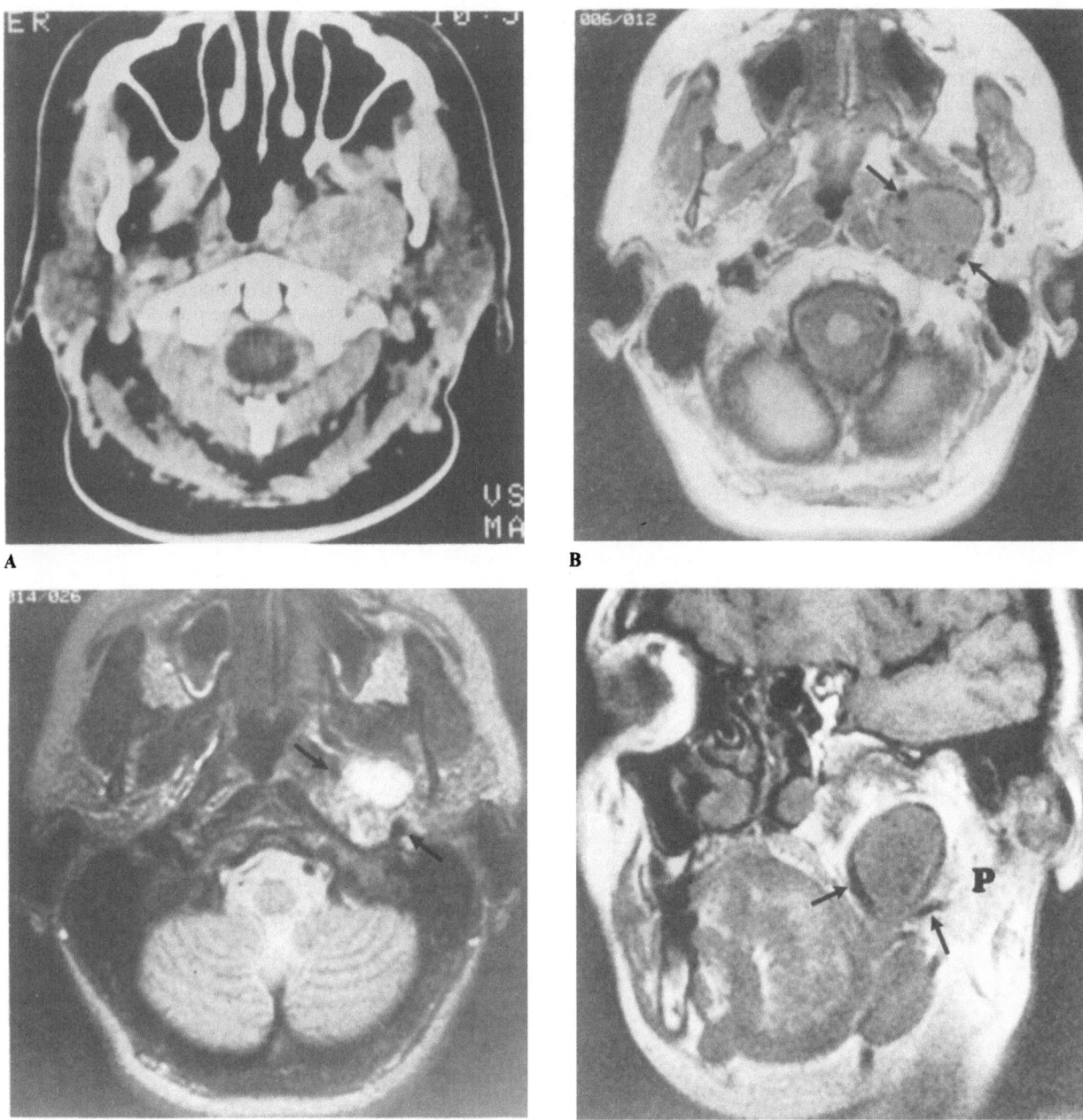

A

B

C

D

Figure 32.(A) *Axial contrast CT section through the lower nasopharynx* shows a homogeneous, oval shaped, sharply delimited, slightly enhancing mass in the left parapharyngeal space. The lesion is adjacent to the deep portion of the left parotid gland and displaces the left lateral pharyngeal wall medially. The tumor encroaches upon the medial pterygoid muscle and lies adjacent to the atlas.

(B & C) *Comparable axial MR images* [(32B) *TR 600/TE 20 − NEX = 2; (32C) TR 2000/TE 80 − NEX= 1. SLT = 0.5 cm*]. A mass of intermediate SI with several foci of low SI is demonstrated in the left parapharyngeal space on the T_1-CW image (Figure 32B), splaying the internal and external carotid vessels (arrows).

The tumor is adjacent to the longus capitis muscle, the medial pterygoid muscle and the deep lobe of the parotid gland, without invasion of the fat anteriorly and posteriorly. On the T_2-CW image (Figure 32C), the mass has high SI, mainly anteriorly with serpiginous channels of low SI, posteriorly. On both images, arrows point to signal voids, representing the internal and external carotid arteries displaced by the mass.

(D) *Oblique coronal MR image (TR 500/TE 20 − NEX = 2; SLT = 0.5 cm)* demonstrates the same mass of intermediate SI splaying vessels (arrows), without evidence of invasion of adjacent structures, especially of the parotid gland (P).

131

I. Parapharyngeal space

enhancement of a suspected vascular tumor is best accomplished with a dynamic scan. If the examination is carried out with a slow infusion (over a period of about ten minutes), enhancement may be only slight and, therefore, fail to differentiate this vascular tumor from other nonvascular lesions, such as mixed tumors, neurogenic tumors (neurilemmoma, neurofibroma) and lymphomas.

MRI depicts the boundaries of the lesion in the parapharyngeal space more clearly than CT. MRI delineates, in addition, the blood vessels without the introduction of contrast material. On the CT examination, the carotid artery merges with the mass and cannot be separated. On MR it appears as a signal void contrasting with the inter-mediate SI mass (Figure 32D). The use of Gadolinium-DTPA may optimally delineate glomus tumors by virtue of increased SI on T_1-CW images [57–58]. Owing to its multiplanar capability, especially coronal views, MR also provides useful information concerning the tumor extent.

Moreover, MR images show signal void areas that represent small tumor vessels, as proved by histology. Serpiginous tubular signal void structures are found on MR in a high percentage of glomus tumors [20]. As a consequence, MR suggested a very vascular lesion even before angiography. The lesion also is surrounded by a low intensity capsule. This is consistent with the pseudocapsules found on histological examination.

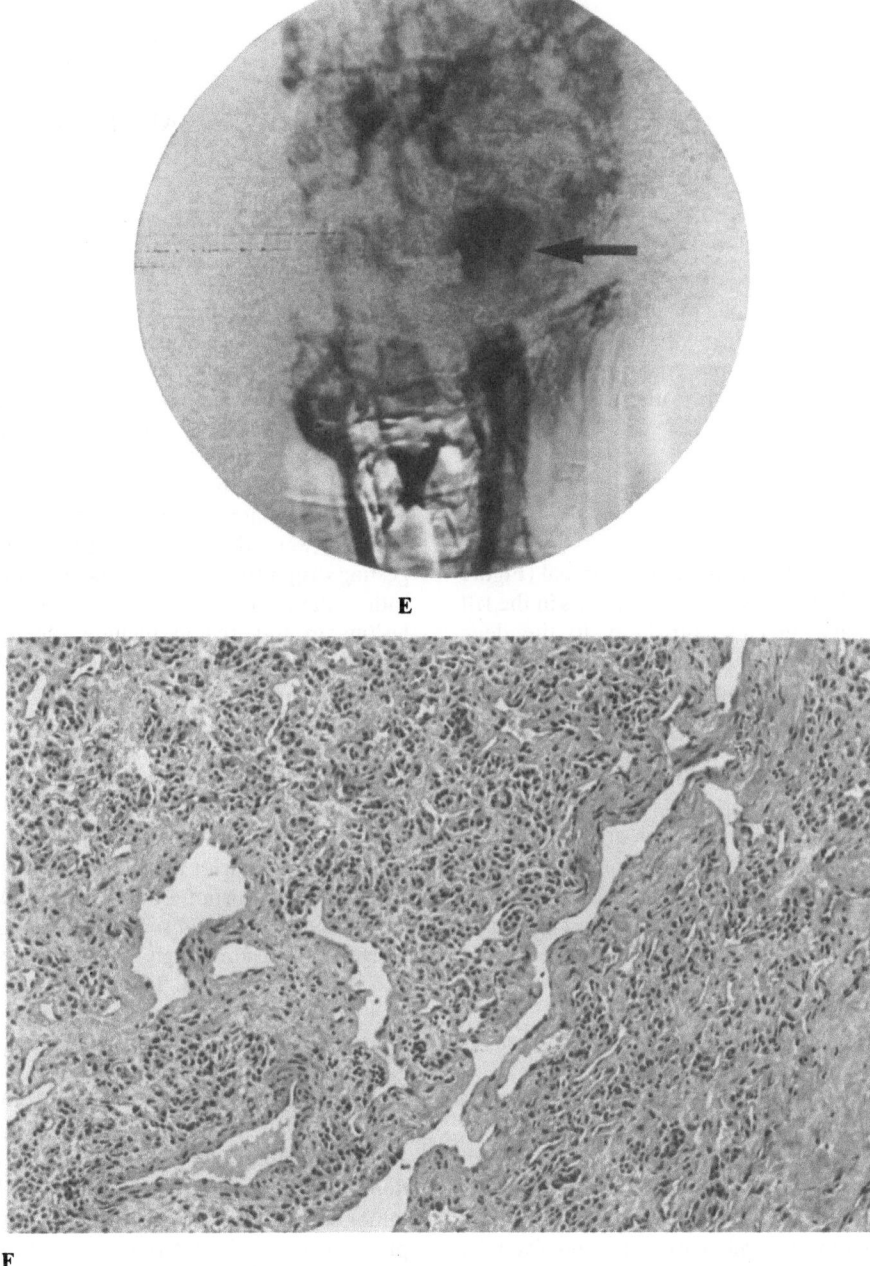

E

F

Figure 32.(E) *Intravenous bilateral angiogram of the carotid system* shows a dense, vascular blush (arrow) in the early capillary phase in the upper third of the neck.

(F) *Photomicrograph of a section through the excised paraganglioma* (125×, hematoxylin and eosin stain). Note the vascular spaces and the balls of cells.

Case 33

MIXED TUMOR OF THE LEFT PARAPHARYNGEAL SPACE

Clinical presentation

A 49 year old female complained of vague neck pain, and was found to have a medial bulge of the lateral oropharyngeal wall with slight medial displacement of the soft palate. The physical examination was otherwise unremarkable.

Radiologic findings

A CT study in the axial (Figure 33A) and coronal (Figure 33C) planes showed a large, nonenhancing mass in the left parapharyngeal space, in close proximity to the deep portion of the left parotid gland with lack of an intervening fat plane. The lesion extended from slightly below the base of skull to the angle of the mandible. MRI, with axial (Figure 33B) and coronal (Figure 33D) views demonstrated a well defined, homogeneous mass of intermediate SI on 'mixed' (T_1- and T_2-CW) images (Figure 33D) and of high SI on T_2-CW images arising from the deep lobe of the left parotid gland without invasion of the adjacent structures. A left common carotid and left external carotid angiogram showed a relatively avascular mass displacing the external carotid artery posteriorly.

Surgical and histological findings

A left total parotidectomy with facial nerve dissection was performed, along with removal of the tumor within the left parapharyngeal space. In conjunction with the parotidectomy, the dissection of the parapharyngeal mass included removal of the posterior belly of the digastric muscle and of the stylohyoid muscle, which were not involved by tumor on pathological examination of the specimen. The main body of the hyoid bone and a superior parotid lymph node were also excised.

The histological examination of the mass revealed a tumor composed of abundant myxoid stroma with occasional nests of ductal cells and myoepithelial cells consistent with pleomorphic adenoma (mixed tumor) (Figure 33E). The excised lymph node was normal.

Comments

The CT study in the axial and coronal planes accurately depicted the site and extent of this lesion. Furthermore, there was no enhancement following the infusion of contrast material, suggestive of a nonvascular lesion. However, detailed assessment of its enhancement features would have required a dynamic CT scan. The coronal sections outline the longitudinal dimension of the lesion and its relationship to the base of skull. There is no fat plane between the lesion and the left parotid gland, suggesting origin from the deep portion of the parotid gland rather than an extraparotid location. Well demarcated lesions in this region include pleomorphic adenomas arising from the deep lobe of the parotid and minor salivary glands, and neurogenic tumors, especially neurilemmomas.

MRI, due to its excellent soft tissue contrast resolution, is superior to CT in defining the boundaries of this mass in relation to the adjacent pterygoid muscles, the lateral pharyngeal wall and the parotid gland. The mass imperceptibly merges with the parotid gland, suggesting origin from the deep portion of the gland. This finding is further strengthened by the absence, on 'mixed' (proton density) images, of a distinct high SI fat plane between the tumor and the parotid gland. The existence of such a fat plane [20] would have been in favor of a minor salivary gland tumor with secondary encroachment upon the parotid gland. The high SI of this mixed tumor on T_2-CW images is consistent with the abundant myxoid stroma (comparable biochemically to a proteinacenous soluton).

Histopathologically, differentiation between a mixed tumor originating in the deep parotid lobe and a mixed tumor arising from the minor salivary glands of the pharyngeal wall is not possible. A minor salivary gland tumor should present as a submucosal mass, and manifest as a pharyngeal, intraluminal growth. However, other large parapharyngeal tumors, including those large masses that arise from the deep portion of the parotid, present in the same manner [59].

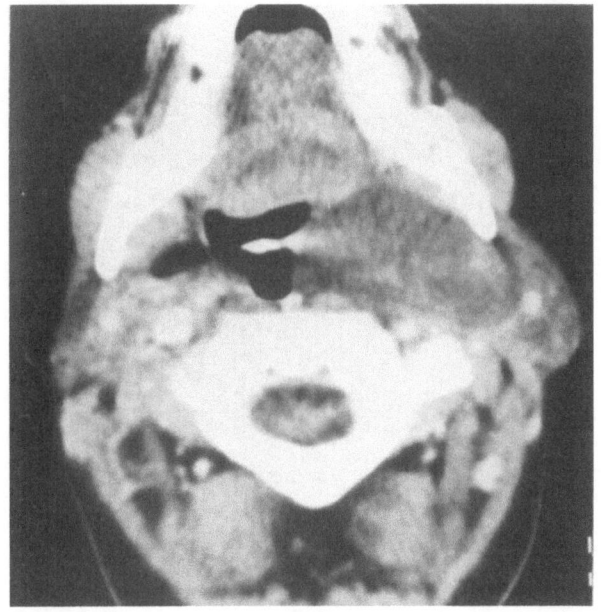

A

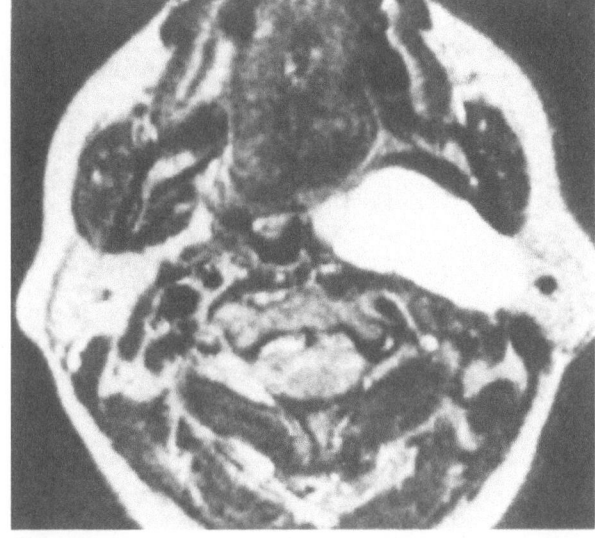

B

C

D

Figure 33.* (A) *Axial contrast CT section at the level of the oropharynx* reveals a large, homogeneous mass that is oval in shape and located within the left parapharyngeal space. The mass has slightly low attenuation values in relation to muscle. The lesion arises from the deep portion of the parotid gland, reaching the lateral pharyngeal wall, which is displaced medially. The lesion extends posteriorly to the cervical spine and anteriorly to the mandible. The soft palate is slightly displaced medially.

(B) *Comparable axial MR projection (TR 2000/TE 80 − NEX = 2; SLT = 0.5 cm)* shows a lobulated mass in the left parapharyngeal space of high SI with a focus of low SI along the medial aspect of the mass, probably representing hemorrhage, subsequent to fine needle aspiration performed through the oropharynx a few weeks earlier. The lesion extends from the parotid gland to the left lateral wall of the oropharynx encroaching upon the medial pterygoid muscle and slightly displacing the soft palate to the right. There is no fatty cleavage between the tumor and parotid gland.

(C) *Coronal contrast CT section at the level of the pharynx* demonstrates a large mass in the parapharyngeal space extending from slightly below the base of skull to the angle of the mandible. Note the medial bulge of the left pharyngeal wall. The lesion is inseparable from the parotid gland. Due to rotation, the left mandible is only partially demonstrated.

(D) *Comparable coronal MR projection (TR 1000/TE 50 − NEX = 1; SLT = 0.5 cm)* demonstrates a well defined mass of intermediate SI projecting into the left naso- and oropharynx. Note the close relationship of the lesion with the normal parotid tissue (p). The base of skull is not involved.

135

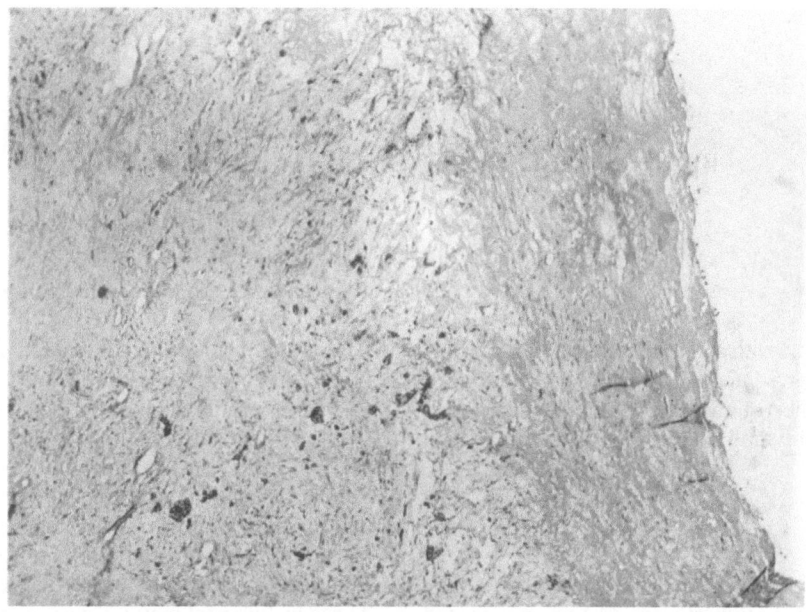

E

Figure 33.*(E) *Photomicrograph of a pleomorphic adenoma in the parapharyngeal space* (45×, hematoxylin and eosin stain). Note abundant myxoid stroma and occasional nests of myoepithelial cells.

* Figure 33 (A–D) appears by courtesy of Dr Greg Shoukimas, West Suburban Imaging Center, Wellesley, Mass., U.S.A.

137

Case 34

BRANCHIAL CLEFT CYST OF THE RIGHT NECK

Clinical presentation

A 27 year old woman with a three month history of high right neck swelling, presented with a 2 to 3 cm ovoid mass at the anterior border of the right sternocleidomastoid muscle. No enlarged lymph nodes were found on clinical examination.

Radiologic findings

A noncontrast axial CT study (Figure 34A) demonstrated an isodense mass, suggestive of a solid lesion, possibly arising from the tail of the right parotid gland.

MRI, with axial (Figures 34B, C, & D) and coronal (Figure 34E) projections revealed a sharply defined mass, with complex MR signal characteristics (Table 3), adjacent to the posteromedial and inferior aspects of the parotid gland. No enlarged lymph nodes were identified. The MR signal characteristics were compatible with a cyst, but not with a solid neoplasm, as suspected on the CT study.

Surgical and histopathological findings

Surgery confirmed the presence of a cystic structure that was distinct from the parotid gland.

Pathological examination of the mass showed a cystic structure, measuring $3 \times 2 \times 1.3$ cm, with a smooth lining and a pink-yellowish fluid composed of proteinaceous debris, desquamated epithelial cells, inflammatory cells, and cholesterol cystals. Histologically, the cyst was lined by stratified squamous epithelium with focal keratinization and was surrounded by a rim of lymphoid tissue. These histological features were consistent with a branchial cleft cyst.

Comments

MR, compared to CT, gave a better characterization and localization of the mass in the neck, confirming the diagnosis of a cyst in an extraparotid location. A solid lesion, as opposed to a cyst, has lower SI on T_2-CW images.

However, the signal characteristics of this mass were unusual for cystic fluid, that usually has high SI on T_2-CW images and low SI on T_1-CW images. These SI variations can be explained by the complex biochemical composition of the fluid. Moreover, the appearance of the high SI structures around the cyst are consistent with lymphoid tissue.

Table 3. MR signal characteristics of various tissues on Figures 34B, C & D.

Tissues	T_1-CW	T_2-CW ($TE = 96$)	GRE ($TE = 30$, $\alpha = 30°$, $TR = 100$)
Fat	Very high	High	Intermediate
Muscle	Intermediate	Intermediate	Intermediate
Water (CSF)	Very low	Very high	Very high*
Lesion	Moderately high	Low	High
Subacute hemorrhage	High	Low	Very low

* Due to flow of unsaturated spins into imaged volume, there is high SI within CSF and blood vessels. Without *flow effect*, CSF would have intermediate SI with this pulse sequence.

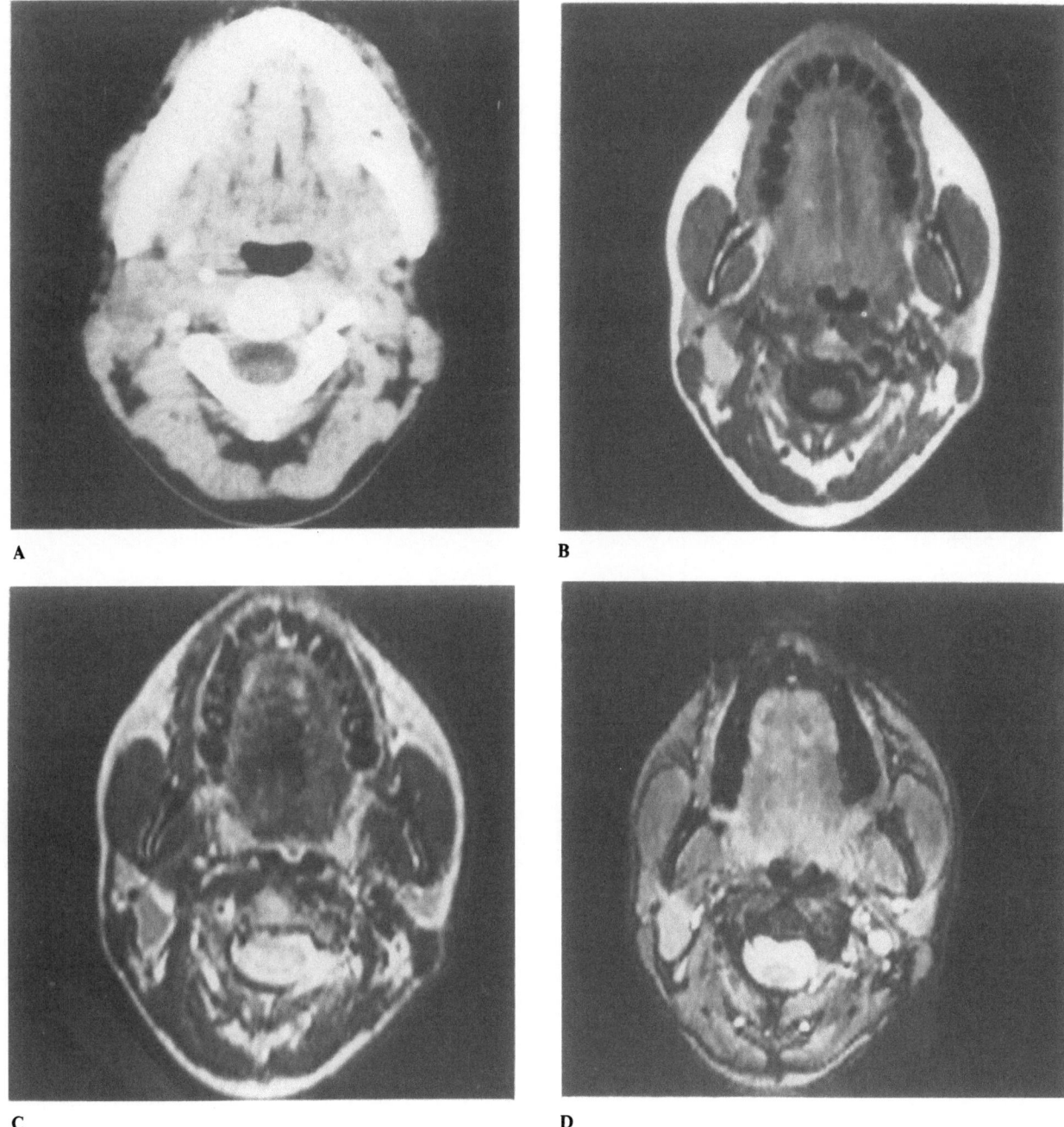

A

B

C

D

Figure 34.(A) *Axial noncontrast CT section at the level of the angle of the mandible* shows a right, isodense oval-shaped, well defined mass of about 3 cm in diameter.
(B, C & D) *Comparable axial MR projections* [(34B) *TR* 350/ *TE* 25 − NEX = 4; (34C) *TR* 2000/*TE* 96 − NEX = 2; (34D) partial saturation gradient echo image (GRE) with low flip angle (α = 30°), *TR* 100/*TE* 30 − NEX = 4. SLT = 0.7 cm]. A well defined mass is visualized medial to the right sternocleidomastoid muscle, adjacent to the inferior aspect of the parotid gland and

the lateral aspect of the scaleni muscles. The SI on the T_1-CW image (Figure 34B) is moderately high, but lower than fat. On the T_2-CW image (Figure 34C), the central portion of the mass has rather low SI with a thickened, irregular high SI wall. The mass has high SI (higher than fat) on the GRE image (Figure 34D). Table 3 shows the MR characteristics of various tissues. No signal abnormality suggestive of infection or malignant neoplasm is noted either in the adjacent fat or muscle or in the adjacent parotid gland.

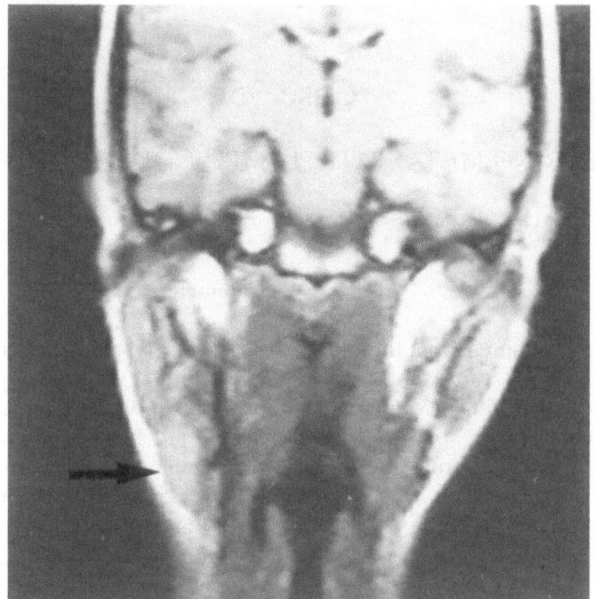

E

Figure 34. (E) *Coronal MR projection at mid-parotid level (TR 300/TE 25 − NEX = 4; SLT = 0.7 cm) shows a moderately high* SI longitudinal mass (arrow) bordering on the inferior aspect of the right parotid gland.

Case 35

CYSTIC-APPEARING METASTATIC LYMPH NODE IN THE RIGHT NECK

Clinical presentation

For six years, an 83 year old man suffered from multiple skin cancers of the face and neck which were excised each time they appeared. He represented with a 3 cm right supraclavicular mass which increased in size to 6 cm within one month. A lesion in the left external auditory canal was also noted.

Radiologic findings

An axial CT study (Figure 35A) showed a large, cystic mass in the right neck beneath the sternocleidomastoid muscle, extending from the level of the mid thyroid cartilage down to the thoracic inlet. No enlarged lymph nodes were seen. The internal jugular vein was not identified.

MRI, with axial (Figure 35B & C) and coronal (Figure 35D) sections, showed a cystic mass that appeared to have irregular walls. Neither flow nor thrombus could be seen in the internal jugular vein. The differential diagnoses were infected branchial cleft cyst or a necrotic metastatic lymph node.

Surgical and histological findings

Malignant cells were found by needle aspiration and the patient underwent a right radical neck dissection. On histopathologic examination, metastatic squamous cell carcinoma was found in four out of eleven normal sized, lymph nodes. The right lower neck specimen contained several matted nodes with a large cavitary area. This cavity (Figure 35E) was lined by keratinized, necrotic squamous cells and surrounded by lymphoid tissue with extranodal tumor extension. The right internal jugular vein was compressed and focally invaded.

The lesion of the external auditory canal was excised, and the histopathological examination revealed an invasive, keratinizing squamous cell carcinoma with focal erosion of the auricular cartilage, as well as a small basal cell carcinoma.

Comments

Metastatic disease in a cervical node with necrosis is a frequent finding, but the appearance as a cystic mass is less common [60]. In this case, the metastatic lymph node manifested as a true cyst that resulted from complete replacement of a few aggregated lymph nodes by tumor (Figure 35E). Peripherally, the compressed lymphoid elements are probably represented by the oblong high SI structures, seen on T_2-CW images (Figure 35C). Well-differentiated (keratinized) squamous cell carcinomas are lesions that may undergo cystification. The desquamated keratin produces inflammatory changes with polymorphonuclear infiltrates. The enzymes of these leukocytes are probably responsible for tissue breakdown, with the ultimate formation of a cystic cavity.

On CT, this cystic appearing necrotic metastatic lymph node is difficult to differentiate from a branchial cleft cyst, although branchial cysts are usually located in the upper neck at the angle of the mandible.

Likewise, MR demonstrates a fluid-filled structure, as evidenced by a high SI on T_2-CW images. The coronal images clearly define the longitudinal extension of this cystic lesion. In order to image the neck from the external auditory canal to the thoracic inlet, in axial sections, the TR used in this MR study for T_1-CW images was slightly longer than usual (550 msec instead of 400–500 msec) and the slice thickness was increased (0.7 cm instead of 0.5 or 0.4 cm) [see page 8, paragraph 2.7].

Additionally, an attempt was made to demonstrate flow in the right internal jugular vein, employing the phenomenon of even echo rephasing [60]. Even echoes of a multiple-spin echo train have higher SI than the odd echoes, since they correct velocity-induced phase error, yielding increased SI within the vascular lumen when compared with the preceding echo. Single-slice gradient echo imaging can also demonstrate flow as unsaturated protons move into the imaged volume. MRI excluded thrombosis of the internal jugular vein. However, it was uncertain whether the vein was compressed, invaded, or absent. The pathological examination of the specimen revealed focal invasion of the vein, resulting in diminished flow and collapse.

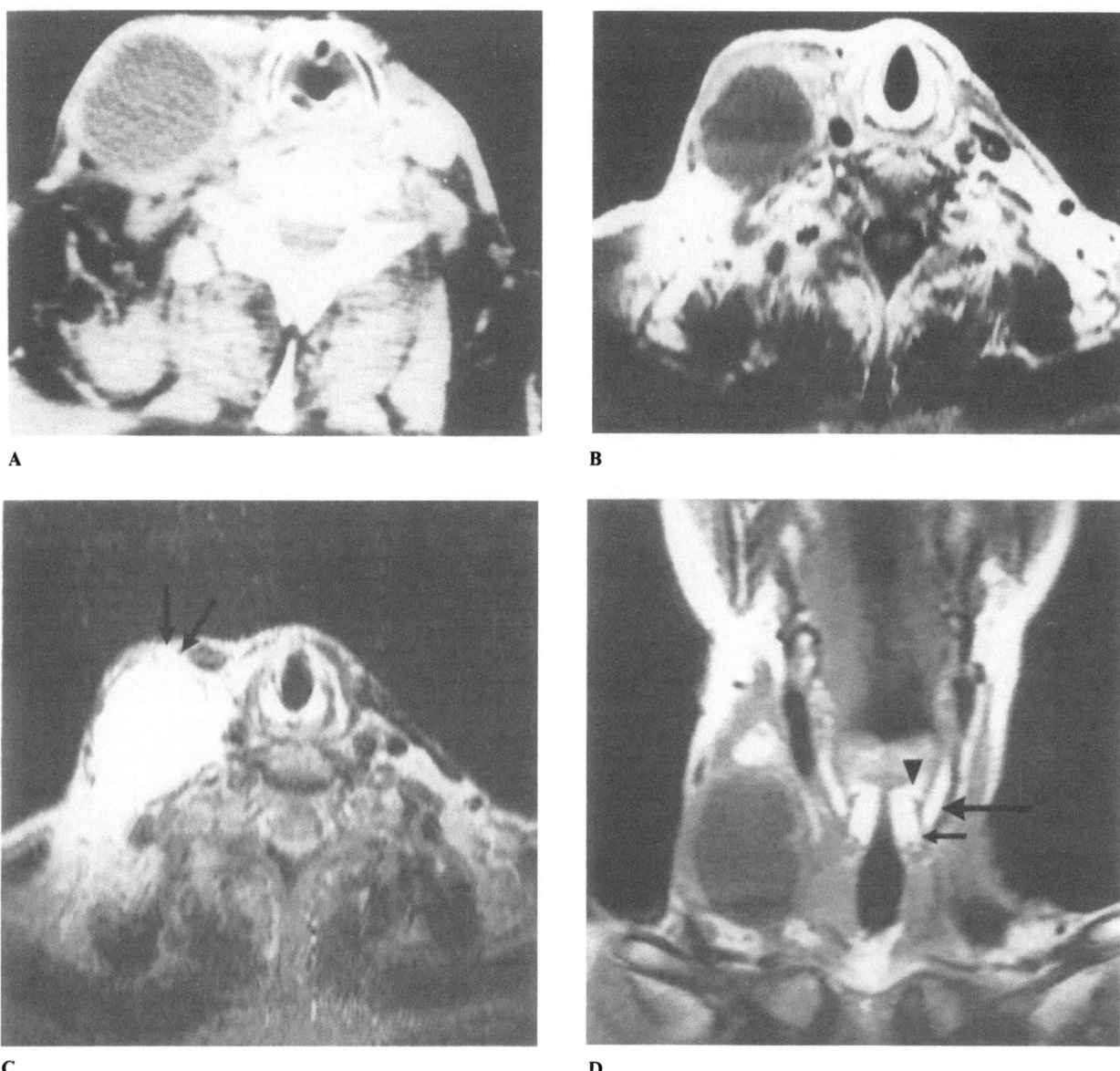

A

B

C

D

Figure 35. (A) *Axial contrast CT through the lower neck* reveals a large, fairly well defined, cystic, thin walled mass with a diameter of about 5 cm. The right internal jugular vein is not visible. The right common carotid artery appears to be in normal position.
(B & C) *Axial MR projections at comparable level* [(35B) *TR 500/TE 21* − NEX = 4; (35C) *TR 2000/TE 90* − NEX = . SLT = 0.7 cm] show a cystic mass in the right neck, as evidenced by a very high SI on the T_2-CW image (Figure 35C). On the right side, only the carotid artery is visualized; whereas on the left side both the common carotid artery and the internal jugular vein are demonstrated. The fluid–fluid level (Figure 35B) probably stems

from a recent needle aspiration, which may have produced some bleeding. The cyst wall cannot be well characterized, due to the limited spatial resolution of MR. Oblong structures of very high SI on the T_2-CW image of very high SI on the T_2-CW image are noted adjacent to the cyst (arrows). These structures are compatible with compressed lymph nodes.
(D) *Coronal MR projection at level of anterior neck* (*TR 550/ TE 21* − NEX = 4; SLT = 0.5 cm). A mass of low SI extends from the mid thyroid cartilage to the fat of the supraclavicular fossa. The larynx at its posterior aspect appears normal; note thyroid (long arrow), cricoid (short arrow), arytenoid (arrowhead) cartilages. No enlarged lymph nodes are identified.

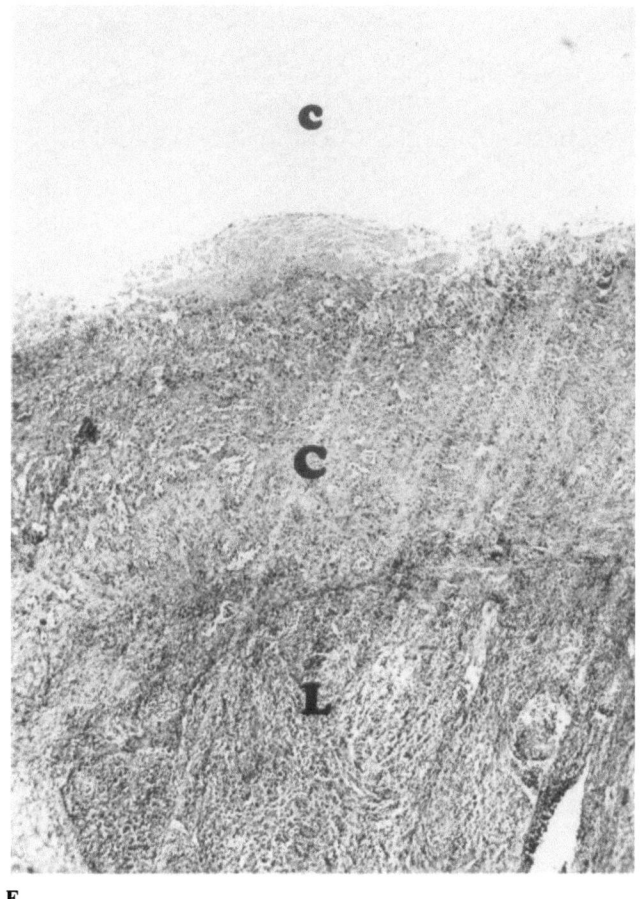

E

Figure 35.(E) *Photomicrograph of a section through the excised neck mass* (30×, hematoxylin and eosin stain) shows a cystic cavity (c) lined by squamous cell carcinoma (C) and lymphoid tissue (L) of confluent nodes.

REFERENCES FOR CHAPTER THREE: CASE PRESENTATIONS

1. Peyster RG, Shapiro MD, Haik BG (1987): Orbital metastasis – Role of magnetic resonance imaging and computed tomography. *Radiol. Clin. North. Am.* 25: 647–667.
2. Som PM, Shapiro MD, Biller HF, et al. (1988): Sinonasal tumors and inflammatory tissues. Differentiation with MR imaging. *Radiology* 167: 803–808.
3. Gomori JM, Grossman RI, Zimmerman RA, et al. (1985): Intracranial hematomas: Imaging by high field MR. *Radiology* 159: 87–93.
4. Maurer HM, Beltangady M, Gehan EA, et al. (1988): The intergroup rhabdomyosarcomas study – 1. *Cancer* 61: 209–220.
5. New PFJ, Rosen BR, Brady TJ et al. (1983): Potential hazards and artifacts of ferromagnetic and nonferromagnetic surgical and dental materials and devices in nuclear magnetic resonance imaging. *Radiology* 147: 139–148.
6. Daniels DL, Pech P, Mark L, et al. (1985): Magnetic resonance imaging of the cavernous sinus. *AJNR* 6: 187–192.
7. Aegerter E, Kirkpatrick JA Jr. (1975): *Orthopedic Diseases*, 4th ed., pp. 167–174. Philadelphia: W. B. Saunders Co.
8. Mitchell DG, Burk DL Jr, Viniski S, et al. (1987): The biophysical basis of tissue contrast in extracranial MR imaging. *AJR* 149: 831–837.
9. Hackney DB, Grossman RI, Zimmerman RA, et al. (1987): Low sensitivity of clinical MR imaging to small changes in the concentration of nonparamagnetic protein. *AJNR* 8: 1003–1008.
10. Gomori JM, Grossman RI, Hackney DB, et al. (1987): Variable appearances of subacute intracranial hematomas on high field spin echo. *AJNR* 8: 1019–1026.
11. Suit H, Griffin T, Almond P, et al. (1984): Particle radiation therapy. *Cancer Treatment Symp.* 1: 147–160.
12. Weber AL (1988): Radiological evaluation of chondrosarcomas of the head and neck region. Presented at the *XI International Congress of Head and Neck Radiology*, 6–11 June 1988, Uppsala, Sweden.
13. Oot RF, Melville GE, New PFJ, Austin-Seymour M, et al. (1988): The role of MR and CT in evaluating clival chordomas and chondrosarcomas. *AJNR* 9: 715–723.
14. Nadol JB Jr., Schuknecht HF (1984): Obliteration of the mastoid in the treatment of tumors of the temporal bone. *Ann. Otol. Rhinol. Laryngol.* 93: 6–12.
15. Hahn SS, Kim JA, Goodchild N, Constable WC (1983): Carcinoma of the middle ear and external auditory canal. *Int. J. Rad. Oncol. Biol. Phys.* 9: 1003–1007.
16. Westesson PL, Katzberg RW, Tallents RH, et al. (1987): Temporomandibular joint: Comparison of MR images with cryosectional anatomy. *Radiology* 164: 59–64.
17. Vogl T, Brunning R, Schedel H, et al. (1988): MR imaging of paragangliomas of the jugular bulb and carotid body: Fast imaging technique and Gd-DTPA. Presented at the *74th Scientific Assembly and Annual Meeting of the Radiological Society of North America*, 27 November–2 December 1988, Chicago, Ill., U.S.A.
18. Glenner GG, Grimley PM (1974): Branchiomeric and intravagal paraganglia. In: Tumors of the extra-adrenal paraganglion system. *Atlas of Tumor Pathology, Fascicle 9*, pp. 17–33. Washington: Armed Forces Institute of Pathology.
19. Michael AS, Mafee MF, Valvassori GE, et al. (1985): Dynamic computed tomography of the head and neck: Differential diagnosis value. *Radiology* 154: 413–419.
20. Som PM, Braun IF, Shapiro MD, et al. (1987): Tumors of the parapharyngeal space and upper neck: MR imaging signal characteristics. *Radiology* 164: 823–829.
21. Paling MR, Black WC, Levin PA, et al. (1987): Tumor invasion of the anterior skull base: a comparison of MR and CT studies. *JCAT* 11: 824–830.
22. Rubinstein LJ (1972): *Tumors of the Central Nervous System. Fascicle 6*, pp. 206–212. Washington: Armed Forces Institute of Pathology.
23. Gentry LR, Jacoby CG, Turski PA, et al. (1987): Cerebellopontine angle-petromastoid mass lesions: Comparative study of diagnosis with MR imaging and CT. *Radiology* 162: 513–520.
24. Mikhael MA, Ciric IS, Wolff AP (1985): Differentiation of cerebellopontine angle neuromas and meningiomas with MR imaging. *JCAT* 9: 852–856.
25. Greenberg JJ, Oot RF, Wismer GL, et al. (1988): Cholesterol granuloma of the petrous apex: MR and CT evaluation. *AJNR* 9: 1205–1214.
26. Sataloff RT, Myers DL, Roberts BR, et al. (1988). Giant cholesterol cysts of the petrous apex. *Arch. Otolaryngol. Head Neck Surg.* 114: 451–453.
27. Griffin C, DeLaPaz R, Enzman D (1987): MR and CT correlation of cholesterol cysts of the petrous apex. *AJNR* 8: 825–829.
28. Steffey DG, DeFilipp GJ, Spera T, et al. (1988): MR imaging of primary epidermoid tumors. *JCAT* 12: 438–440.
29. Thedinger B, Montgomery WW (1989): Radiographic diagnosis, surgical treatment and long term followup of cholesterol granulomas of the petrous apex. Presented at the *American Laryngological, Rhino-*

Case presentations

logical and Otological Society Inc. (Eastern Section) Meeting, 26 January 1989, Toronto, Canada.

30. Teresi L, Lufkin RB, Wortham DG, et al. (1987): Parotid masses by MR imaging. Radiology 163: 405–409.
31. Mandelblatt SM, Braun IF, Davis PC, et al. (1987): Parotid masses: MR imaging. Radiology 163: 411–414.
32. Mikulis DJ, Chisin R, Wismer GL, et al. (1989). Phase contrast imaging of the parotid region. AJNR 10: 157–164.
33. Buxton RB, Edelman RE, Rosen BR, et al. (1987): Contrast in rapid MR imaging – T_1- and T_2-weighted imaging. JCAT 11: 7–16.
34. Teresi L, Lufkin R, Wortham D, et al. (1987): MR imaging of the intratemporal facial nerve by using surface coils. AJR 148: 589–594.
35. Mooyaart EL, Kamman RL, Vermey et al. (1987): Magnetic resonance imaging, a potential application to characterization of parotid tumors. Presented at the 6th annual meeting of the Society of Magnetic Resonance in Medicine, 17–21 August 1987. New York.
36. Batsakis JG (1979): Tumors of the Head and Neck – Clinical and Pathological Considerations, pp. 54–57. Baltimore: Williams and Wilkins Co.
37. Achray TH, Lucas RB (1974): Tumors of the Major Salivary Glands, 52pp. Washington: Armed Forces Institute of Pathology.
38. Blanck C, Eneroth CM, Jakobsson PA (1970): Oncocytoma of the parotid gland: Neoplasm or nodular hyperplasia. Cancer 25: 919–925.
39. Wismer GL, Rosen BR, Buxton RB, et al. (1987): Chemical shift imaging of bone marrow: Preliminary experience. AJR 145: 1031–1037.
40. Corid RL, Sciubba JJ, Brannon RB, et al. (1982): Epithelial-myoepithelial carcinoma of intercalated duct origin: A clinicopathologic and ultrastructural assessment of sixteen cases. Oral Surg. 53: 280–287.
41. Som PM, Scherl MP, Rao VM, et al. (1986): Rare presentations of ordinary lipomas of the head and neck: A review. AJNR 7: 657–664.
42. Korentager R, Noyek AM, Chapnik JS, et al. (1988): Lipoma and liposarcoma of the parotid gland: High resolution preoperative imaging diagnosis. Laryngoscope 98: 967–971.
43. Teresi LM, Lufkin RB, Vinuela F, et al. (1987): MR imaging of the nasopharynx and floor of the middle cranial fossa, Part II: Malignant tumors. Radiology 164: 817–821.
44. Brown AP, Urie MM, Chisin R, et al. (1989): Proton therapy for carcinoma of the nasopharynx: A study in comparative treatment planning. Int. J. Rad. Oncol., Biol., Phys. 16: 1607–1614.
45. Chisin R, Buxton RB, Beaulieu PA, et al. (1989): Preliminary results with low flip angle spin-echo imaging: applications to the head and neck. AJNR 10: 719–724.
46. Vogl T, Bruning R, Grevers G, et al. (1988): MR imaging of the oropharynx and tongue: Comparison of plain and Gd-DTPA studies. JCAT 12: 427–433.
47. Ervin TJ, Clark JR, Weichselbaum RR, et al. (1987): An analysis of induction and adjuvant chemotherapy in the multidisciplinary treatment of squamous cell carcinoma of the head and neck. J. Clin. Otol. 5: 10–20.
48. Weber AL. Personal communication.
49. Lufkin RB, Wortham DG, Dietrich RB, et al. (1986): Tongue and oropharynx: Findings on MR imaging. Radiology 161: 69–75.
50. Som PM (1987): Lymph nodes of the neck. Radiology 165: 593–600.
51. Coakley JF (1985): Primary oat cell carcinoma of the larynx. J. Laryngol. Otol. 99: 301–303.
52. Lufkin RB, Hanafee W, Wortham D, et al. (1986): Larynx and hypopharynx: MR imaging with surface coils. Radiology 158: 747–754.
53. Edelman RR, Stark DD, Saini S. et al. (1986): Oblique planes of section in MR imaging. Radiology 159: 807–810.
54. Gould VE, Dardi LE, Memoli VA, et al. (1980): Neuroendocrine carcinomas of the skin. Light microscope, ultrastructural and immunohistochemical analysis. Ultrastruct. Pathol. 1: 499–509.
55. Glazer HS, Lee JKT, Levitt RG, et al. (1985): Radiation fibrosis: differentiation from recurrent tumor by MR imaging. Radiology 156: 721–726.
56. Ebner F, Kressel HY, Mintz MC, et al. (1988): Tumor recurrence versus fibrosis in the female pelvis: Differentiation with MR imaging at 1.5 T. Radiology 166: 333–340.
57. Breger RK, Papke RA, Pojunas KW, et al. (1987): Benign extra-axial tumors: Contrast enhancement with Gd-DTPA. Radiology 163: 427–429.
58. Haughton VM, Rimm AA, Czervionke LF, et al. (1988): Sensitivity of Gd-DTPA: Enhanced MR imaging of benign extra-axial tumors. Radiology 166: 929–933.
59. Goodman ML (1988). Personal communication.
60. Micheau C, Cachin Y, Caillou B (1974): Cystic metastases in the neck revealing occult carcinoma of the tonsil. A report of six cases. Cancer 33: 228–233.
61. Waluch W, Bradley WG (1984): NMR even echo rephasing in slow laminar flow. JCAT 8: 594–598.

CHAPTER FOUR

MRI strategy in evaluating head and neck tumors

4.1 Introduction

MRI has changed head and neck imaging strategy [1] and has replaced computed tomography (CT) as the radiologic study of choice for some of the extracranial head and neck lesions [2]. MR has the advantage over CT by virtue of its multiplanar imaging capability and its wider range of tissue contrast resolution. Another advantage is the lack of ionizing radiation. Moreover, there is no beam hardening artifact (as seen on the CT images) from dental amalgam and the skull base, including the posterior fossa, and foramen magnum. However, ferromagnetic dental cavity fillings can disturb the magnetic field and degrade the MR image. Due to the superior soft tissue contrast, MRI can also demonstrate vascular anatomy in patients in whom intravenous contrast material cannot be administered.

When compared with CT, MRI has a slightly decreased spatial resolution, suboptimal bone resolution, and a much longer acquisition time, especially in the head and neck where imaging in two or three orthogonal planes is often required.

4.2 Optimum MR imaging parameters

The use of a head coil and a surface coil are necessary in order to improve the S/N ratio, which allows a decrease in the voxel size (the key to improved spatial resolution). A head coil is optimally used for any pathology that does not extend below the level of the tongue. Surface coils, which are available for imaging of the orbits and temporomandibular joints [3], are also very helpful for neck imaging [4].

In a judicious imaging protocol, imaging planes and pulse sequences have to be tailored to each case. Any MR examination should take full advantage of MRI multiplanar imaging capability, and images in at least two orthogonal planes should be obtained. In addition to the three orthogonal planes, oblique planes [5] should also be used in neck imaging. Coronal views allow visualization of the neck structures, including the lymph nodes and vessels, and their relationship to the spine, especially the intervertebral foramina. Furthermore, on coronal views, the pharynx, trachea and thyroid gland can be well depicted.

The pulse sequences utilized include (besides the usual spin echo (SE) sequences) phase contrast imaging for the parotid region [6], using either Dixon's method of chemical shift imaging or partial saturation techniques, with the MR signal read as a 'gradient echo' (GRE); this last pulse sequence being a fast imaging technique. Fast imaging can also be obtained by using a low flip angle double SE technique [7]. Additionally, GRE techniques are used in conjunction with paramagnetic contrast media agents, especially for tongue imaging [8].

Before embarking on a clinical MRI study, a decision should be made concerning the anatomic area to be studied, the optimal S/N ratio, and the desired spatial resolution. These factors, in turn, will determine the matrix size and the slice thickness.

The pathologic process should be evaluated with both T_1- and T_2-CW images to determine the extent and characteristics of the lesion. As an example, hemorrhage can only be distinguished from other tissues if more than one pulse sequence is used. T_1-CW images are best for separating tumor from higher SI fat. T_2-CW images are most helpful in separating tumor or lymph nodes from the relatively lower SI muscle; including delineation of intramuscular pathology (Figure 36). T_2-CW images are also valuable for determining the boundary between the often intermediate SI tumors and the high SI inflammation or blocked secretions commonly associated with paranasal sinus malignancies [9].

Moreover, T_1- and T_2-CW images provide tissue characterization in a small number of lesions, espe-

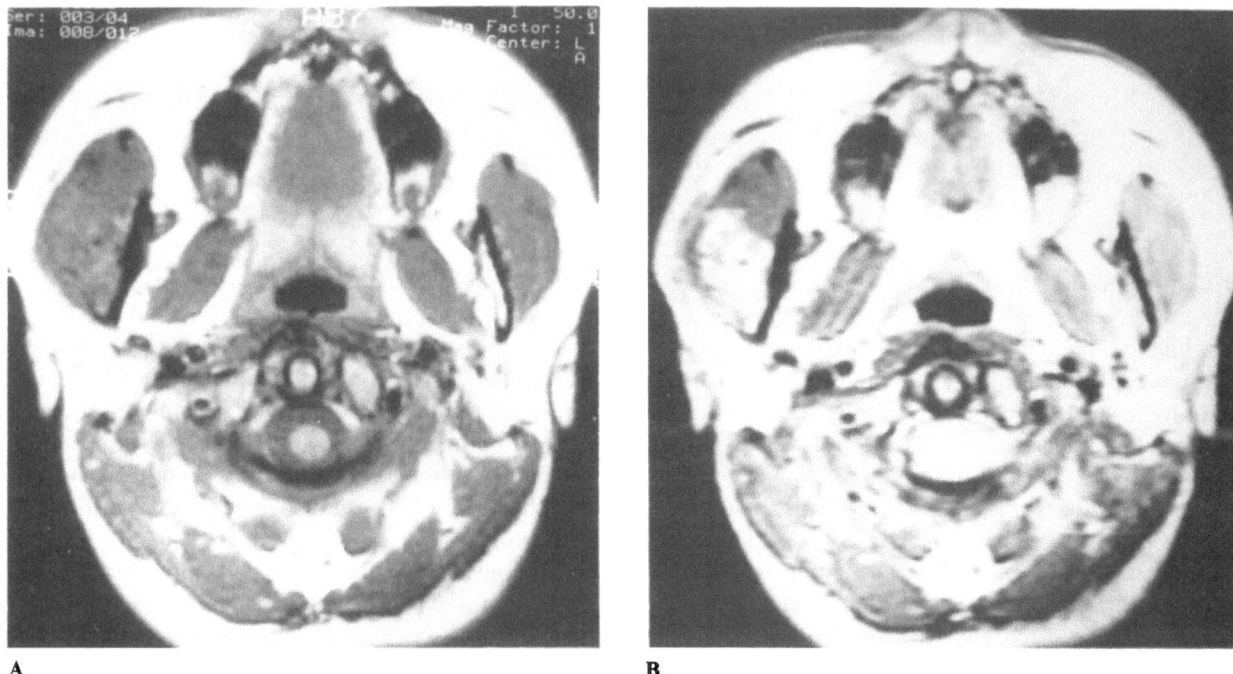

A   B

Figure 36. Axial T_1- (**A**) and T_2 (**B**) CW images show an enlarged right masseter muscle. The pathology (high SI) is demonstrated on the T_2-CW image and contrasts with the muscle that has a lower SI. The lesion was histologically proven to be a lymphangioma. [Fig. 36A & B are reproduced with permission from Chisin R, Fabian R, Weber AL, et al. (1988), MR imaging of a lymphangioma involving the masseter muscle. *JCAT* 12 (4): 690–692.]

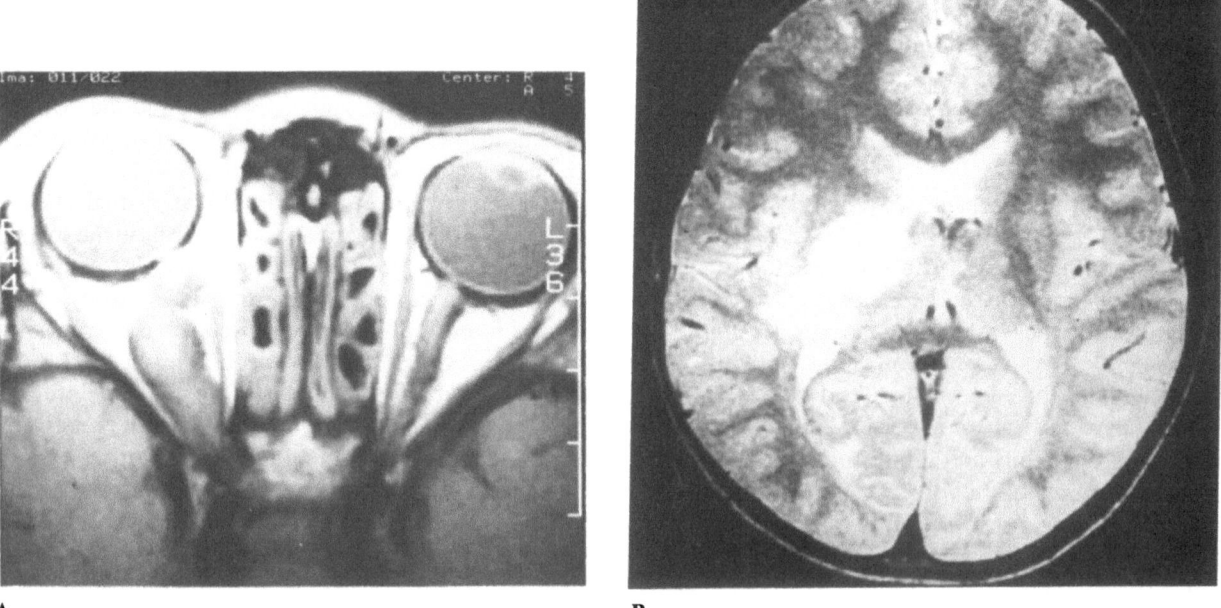

A   B

Figure 37. Axial (**A**) proton density-CW image at the level of the orbits, and (**B**) T_2-CW image at the level above the chiasma, showing an optic nerve glioma. Note enlargement and turtuosity of right optic nerve on Figure 37 (A). Involvement of the right optic tract is characterized by high SI on the T_2-CW image. [Fig. 37A & B appear by courtesy of Dr Gary Stimac, North Shore Magnetic Imaging Center, Peabody, Mass., U.S.A.].

150

cially those containing predominantly fat or fibrous tissue (lipoma, fibrous dysplasia, and occasionally, recurrent tumor in post treatment fibrosis) [10–12].

4.3 MR and head and neck imaging, according to anatomic areas

Because of the variety of anatomic regions of the extracranial head and neck, we will discuss MR imaging strategy by anatomic areas.

Pathology of the orbits, thyroid and parathyroid diseases will only be briefly addressed; and temporomandibular joint imaging is beyond the scope of this book.

4.3.1 Orbital regions

MRI has rapidly become an important imaging technique [13] in the evaluation of orbital lesions, providing both anatomic information and, in some cases, specific tissue characterization (e.g. melanotic melanomas in the appropriate age group).

Axial and coronal projections are mandatory. Direct sagittal images can demonstrate the entire optic nerve (intraorbital, intracanalicular, and intracranial portions).

MRI gives an excellent outline of the lens. Melanotic melanomas are well displayed, because of the paramagnetic effect of melanin, and can also be separated from the frequently associated subretinal fluid collections. Intraorbital optic gliomas and chiasmatic involvement can be detected on T_1-CW images, while gliomas of the optic tract and optic radiation are optimally visualized on T_2-CW images (Figure 37). In case of suspected bone involvement or lesions arising from bone, CT is mandatory for a detailed assessment. As a result, MR and CT are complementary imaging modalities for orbital pathology.

4.3.2 Temporal bone/base of skull

MRI is the modality of choice for evaluating neoplasms of the cerebellopontine angle [14]. MR thin sections and the application of surface coils reliably detect even intracanalicular acoustic tumors [15–16]. The sensitivity in the detection of tumors is further increased by the use of Gadolinium-DTPA [17].

CT remains the study of choice for inflammatory disease and cholesteatoma of the middle ear and mastoid air cells.

However, for tumors of the temporal bone, CT

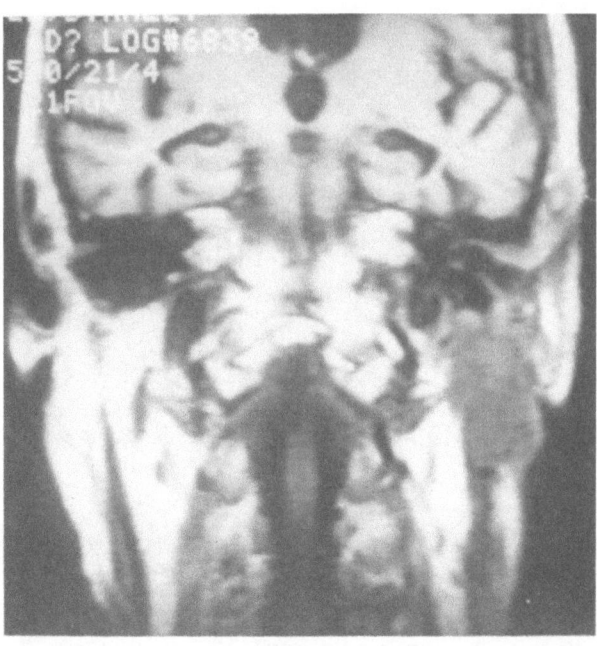

Figure 38. Coronal T_1-CW image showing the neck extension of a squamous cell carcinoma arising in the left temporal bone. Tumor is indicated by intermediate SI. Note obliteration of fat planes.

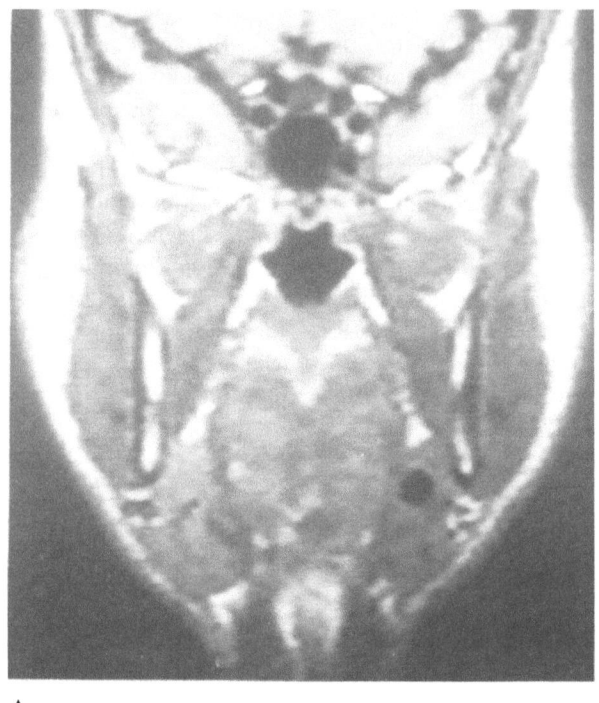

A

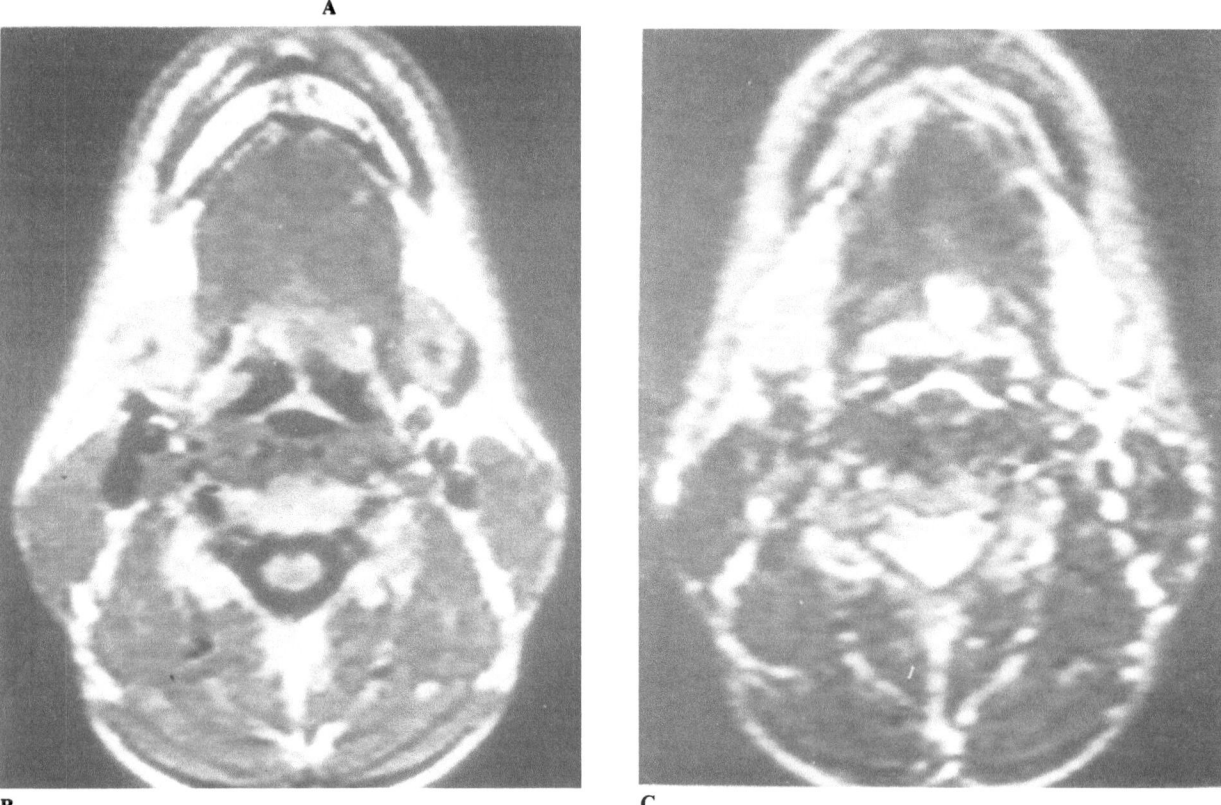

B   C

Figure 39. (A) Coronal T_1-CW image shows the left submandibular gland to be smaller than the right gland with a lower SI and a fairly localized area of signal void corresponding to a stone. (B) Axial T_1-CW image at the level of the glossoepiglottic fold confirmed these findings. (C) Axial T_2-CW image at the same level shows high SI in the left submandibular gland, consistent with high water content of inflammation, secondary to the presence of a stone. Note high SI of lingual tonsil.

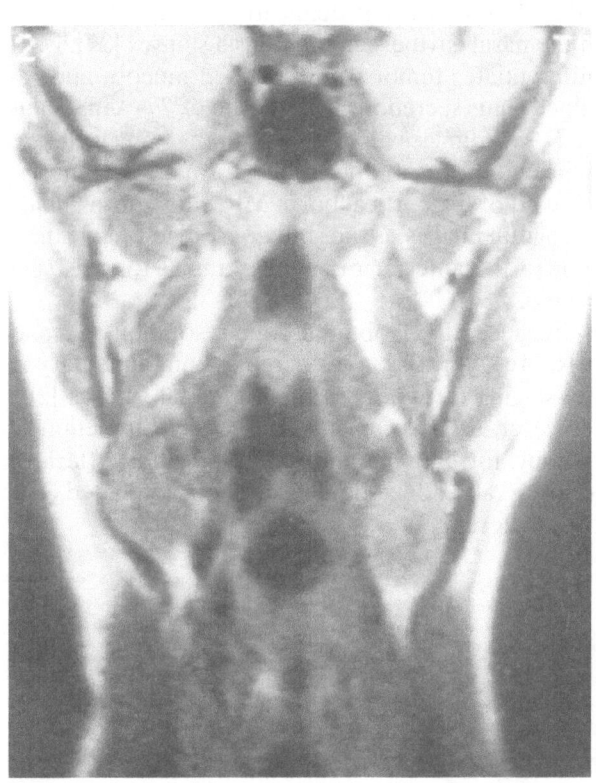

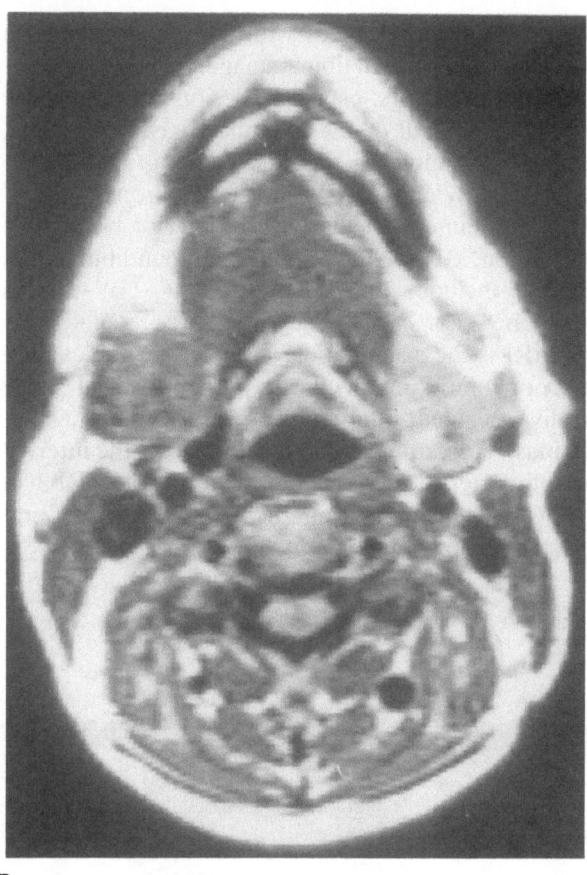

A   **B**

Figure 40. Coronal (**A**) and axial (**B**) T_1-CW images demonstrate a slightly enlarged right submandibular gland with lower SI than the left gland (the same SI pattern was also displayed on T_2-CW images, not shown). Biopsy proved focal, lobular, acute and chronic inflammatory fibrosis in the right gland.

and MRI play a complementary role. MR coronal and sagittal images best detail the intracranial and extracranial extent of the tumor (Figure 38). High resolution CT reveals bone detail, which may be needed in the evaluation of bone destruction, primary bone disease, or congenital malformations. The evaluation of facial nerve tumors benefits from both modalities. Axial, coronal and sagittal MR images, obtained with surface coils, are helpful in visualizing the entire course of the facial nerve [18]. Skull base lesions and cavernous sinus invasion are preferably evaluated by MRI [19, 20], using CT only for detailed assessment of bone abnormalities. Gadolinium-DTPA administration may define some lesions to better advantage, due to tumor enhancement [21].

4.3.3 Salivary glands – Parapharyngeal space

MRI has replaced CT for the evaluation of the majority of tumors in the major salivary glands [22, 23]. However, contrast CT is a more reasonable choice for demonstrating stones, inflammatory masses, and abscesses [24].

The detection of mass lesions in the parotid gland is maximized through the use of both standard SE and phase contrast techniques [6]. The latter can distinguish lesions which are isointense to the normal parotid parenchyma on standard SE imaging. The parotid gland should be screened initially, with a standard T_1-CW SE sequence which, in most cases, detects the lesion. If the lesion clearly demonstrates lower SI than the parotid tissue, a T_2-CW phase contrast acquisition (GRE) will optimize the tissue/lesion contrast. If the lesion is isointense with the parotid tissue, then a T_1-CW phase contrast acquisition (Dixon's method of chemical shift imaging) should provide better contrast. Furthermore, the 'GRE pulse sequences' can be performed, as needed, in place of standard T_2-CW SE sequences to obtain targeted slices with T_2-CW information with significant reduction in imaging time.

In large tumors, especially lesions bordering on the base of skull or the parapharyngeal space [25], the MR examination should include, in addition to axial T_1-CW and T_2-CW-images, a coronal T_1-CW view to define the superior and inferior borders of the lesion. MR evaluation of the submandibular area should include coronal and axial T_1-CW images with one set of T_2-CW images (Figures 39 & 40).

MRI is the examination of choice for the evaluation of tumors involving the parapharyngeal space (salivary gland tumors, neuromas and paragangliomas). According to some authors [26] the internal carotid artery, which is better identified on MRI than on CT is displaced anteriorly by neuromas and posteriorly by salivary lesions.

4.3.4 Paranasal sinuses

MRI allows excellent delineation of tumors arising in the nasal cavities and paranasal sinuses [27]. MRI differentiates tumor from inflamed mucosa and retained sinus secretions with the aid of T_1 - and, mainly, T_2-CW images [9]. Erosions of the bony walls are indicated by the absence of the normally present signal void of the cortical bone. MR, with coronal and/or sagittal images, is the study of choice when extension to the anterior or middle cranial fossa is suspected.

Because of CT optimal bone resolution, CT and MRI are still widely considered as complimentary in the staging of tumors in the paranasal sinuses [28]. However, MRI is replacing CT after completion of therapy, for baseline and follow up studies (lack of ionizing radiation and no intravenous iodinated contrast material).

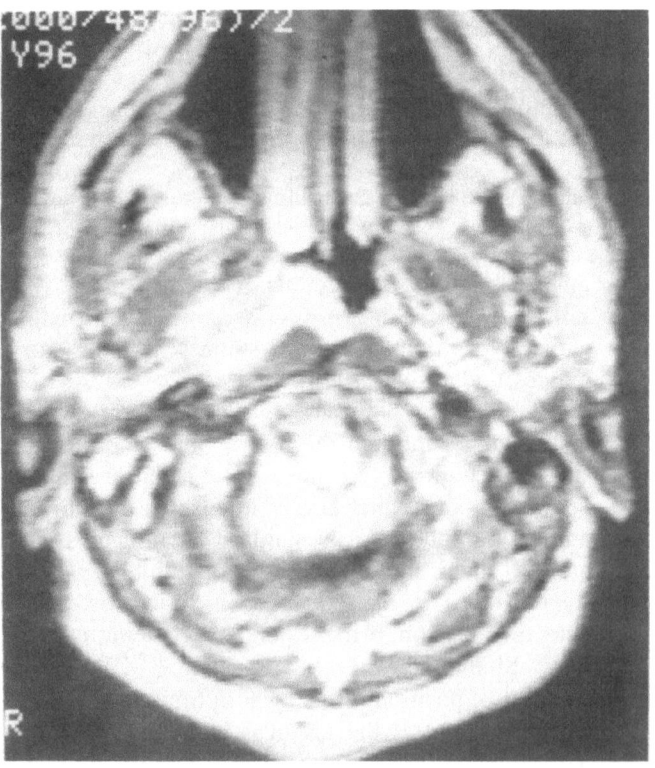 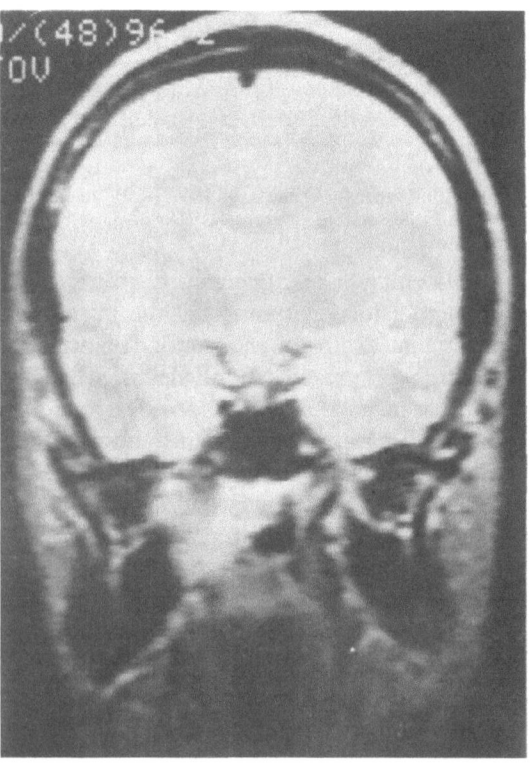

A   B

Figure 41. (**A**) Axial mildly T_2-CW (left) and (**B**) coronal T_2-CW (right) images show clinically unexpected extension of a nasopharyngeal carcinoma into the right parapharyngeal space and right pterygoid muscles. [Fig. 41A & B are reproduced with permission from Brown AP, Urie MM, Chisin R, et al. (1989). Proton therapy for carcinoma of the nasopharynx: A study in comparative treatment planning. *Int. J. Radiat., Oncol., Biol., & Phys.* 16: 1607–1614.]

4.3.5 Nasopharynx

The nasopharynx is a difficult area to visualize on clinical examination. The MR examination is therefore very valuable and should be utilized for tumor detection and evaluation of extent [28].

Axial, coronal, and sagittal views are essential in order to assess craniocaudal and anteroposterior extension of tumors in the nasopharynx. The sagittal views should include all sagittal and parasagittal midline structures encompassing the area between both foramina lacera [2]. Coronal views should also cover the anatomic region from the posterior third of the ethmoid to the anterior border of the foramen magnum.

Axial sections should image the region from the soft palate to the skull base, including the sella and the floor of the middle cranial fossa. T_2-CW images are valuable, since they give a better differentiation between tumor and the soft tissues (prevertebral muscles or parapharyngeal space) than the T_1-CW images (Figure 41).

MRI is superior to CT in imaging the nasopharynx and parapharyngeal space, since the intracranial and extracranial soft tissue components of tumors are better delineated on the MR images [30, 31]. MRI is also a useful adjunct modality to CT for defining the tumor volume [32] to be irradiated (most malignancies of the nasopharynx are squamous cell carcinomas and are irradiated). Although pathologic changes in cortical bone are generally considered to be optimally illustrated by CT, tumor infiltration of bone marrow is more reliably detected with MRI. Thus, CT and MRI are equivalent in assessing erosion of the base of the skull by nasopharyngeal carcinomas. MRI, by combining excellent soft tissue contrast and bone evaluation, is the imaging technique of choice for evaluating the nasopharynx.

MR, is also valuable for the diagnosis and follow-up examinations of juvenile angiofibroma. In this disease, long term follow-up is required to detect early recurrence. Since the tumor occurs in young patients, MR eliminates frequent radiation exposure (resulting from repeated CT examinations). Moreover, in this vascular lesion, low SI areas, due to rapid flow, may be visible [2].

4.3.6 Oropharynx and oral cavity

In the evaluation of tongue masses, the aim is to determine the tumor location, extent and the midline crossing.

Axial sections, which are preferred in establishing the extent of the infiltration across the midline, should include the soft palate and the pre-epiglottic space of the larynx. Sagittal T_1-CW images, which depict the midline structures to best advantage, show posterior spread to the vallecula in carcinomas of the posterior third of the tongue. Combined coronal and sagittal views allow a detailed visualization of the intrinsic tongue musculature – a clear advantage over CT [33].

The musculature of the tongue has a relatively low SI on both T_1- and T_2-CW images. Tumors that have a similar low SI on T_1-CW images may remain undetected, but on T_2-CW images may display an intermediate or high SI, which will then be contrasted against the lower SI muscle. Therefore, T_2-CW images are very valuable in tongue imaging. The detection rate and accurate localization have been significantly improved with the use of Gadolinium-DTPA, used in conjunction with fast imaging (GRE). This technique produces enhancement of the tumor on the T_1-CW images and decreases imaging time, thereby, reducing motion artifact coming from the tongue [8].

The imaging strategy of tonsillar fossa lesions is similar, requiring mainly axial and coronal images. Squamous cell carcinomas of the retromolar trigone, although readily visible and palpable, necessitate imaging studies to determine infiltration into adjacent areas. If mandibular invasion is suspected, CT is still utilized more than MR for ruling out bone involvement, especially with thin 2 mm sections.

4.3.7 Larynx, hypopharynx, and neck

Strategy for laryngeal imaging must ideally include high spatial resolution, axial and coronal images supplemented by axial images of the entire neck from the external auditory canal down to the thoracic inlet. High sensitivity, specially designed neck coils that provide superior S/N ratio, and allow for better spatial resolution are extremely helfpul [4]. Imaging planes should be angulated, in order to be in the axis of the glottis for axial sections, and in the

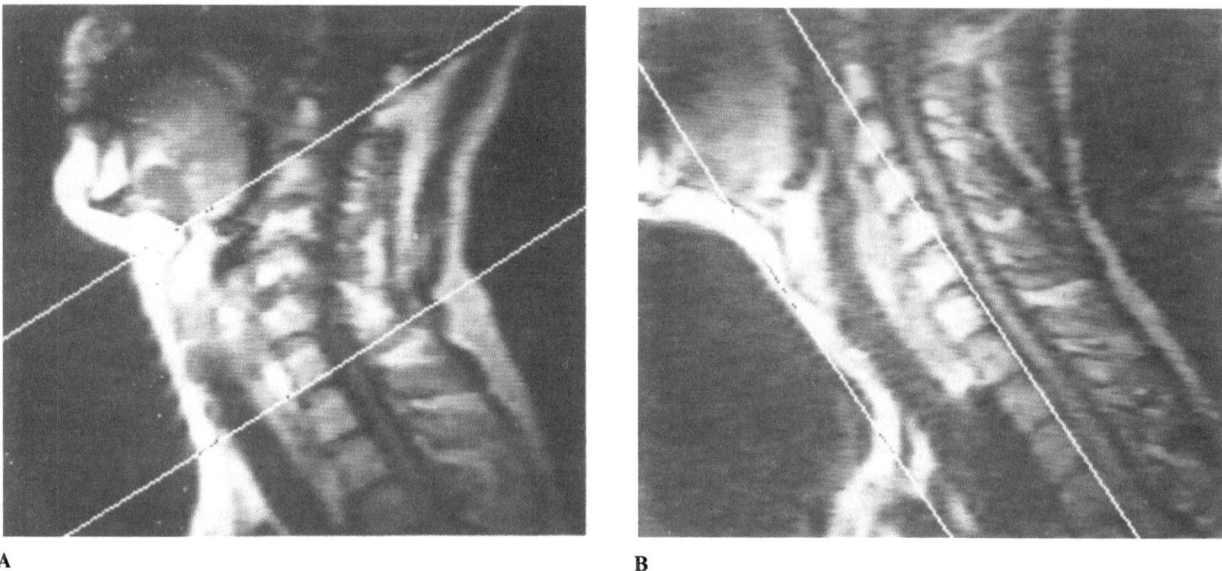

A   **B**

Figure 42.(A) Illustration of angulated axial MR section which is parallel with the plane of the vocal cords. MR plane section is indicated by cursor lines. **(B)** Display of angulated coronal plane used to image the larynx, trachea, hypopharynx. MR section plane is indicted by cursor lines.

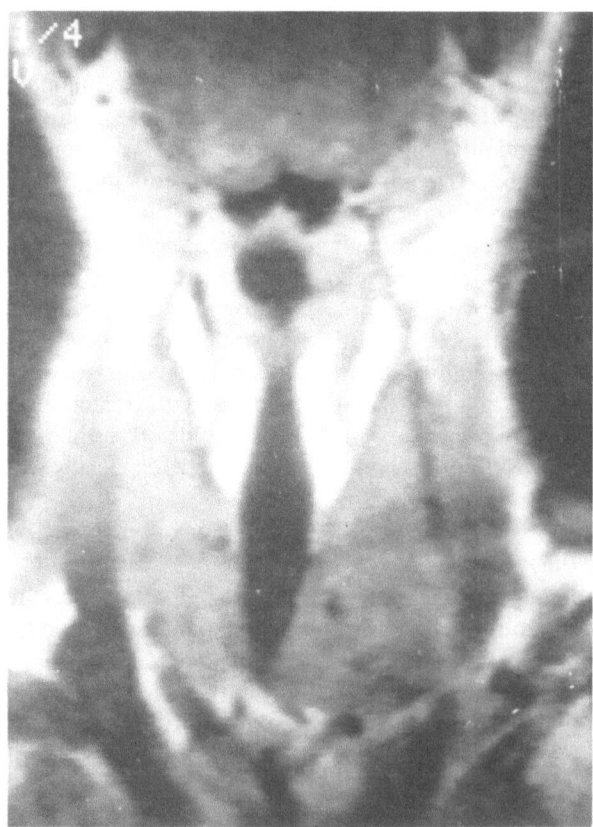

Figure 43. Coronal T_1-CW image shows a squamous cell carcinoma involving the left aryepiglottic fold and the left pyriform fossa. Note the air in the right pyriform sinus.

axis of the laryngotracheal airway for coronal sections [5] (Figure 42).

T_1-CW images maximize contrast between intermediate SI tumors and the fairly high SI of areolar tissue in the paralaryngeal space and the high SI fat in the pre-epiglottic space.

Coronal images help to define the cranio-caudal extension of the tumors (Figure 43). Axial and coronal images depict the anatomy of the aryepiglottic folds, pyriform sinuses, false cords, laryngeal ventricles, true cords, and subglottic space, paralaryngeal space, and thyroid cartilaginous structures. Sagittal images are optimally used in the evaluation of midline structures, such as the pre-epiglottic space and the anterior and posterior commissures. Extension of supraglottic tumors to the vallecular area and tongue is also best evaluated with sagittal views.

MRI does not seem to be more accurate than CT for evaluating subtle invasion of the cartilaginous structures [34]. It is sometimes difficult to assess the thyroid cartilage, since it appears as a discontinuous high SI structure, probably related to its variable calcification–ossification.

Therefore, MR of the larynx is equivalent to CT for tumor staging, but has superior soft tissue contrast and the capability of obtaining direct coronal and sagittal images [35]. However, one other disad-

vantage of MR imaging of the larynx, at the present moment, is the length of time necessary for examinations.

The strategy for hypopharyngeal MR imaging is similar and uses mainly, axial and coronal views.

High resolution images of the thyroid gland can be obtained with surface coils [36, 37]. Cross-axial imaging seems to be the most helpful, but sagittal projections can clearly demonstrate the retrosternal and intrathoracic extension of a goiter (Figure 44). Follicular adenomas, with central hemorrhage and hemorrhagic cyst, show high SI on T_1-CW images. Cystic colloid nodules have high SI on both T_1- and T_2-CW images. Carcinomas have variable MR appearances and are not easily differentiated from other lesions [36, 37]. Multinodular goiters also have variable SI, depending on the tissue composition (Figure 45). Small lesions of the thyroid are best evaluated by ultrasound, while MRI of the thyroid gland yields significant information for large tumors.

The detection of parathyroid abnormalites, especially adenomas, with high resolution MRI compares favorably with other imaging modalities, such as ultrasound and scintigraphy with thallium/technetium pertechnetate [35].

The detection of abnormal lymph nodes in the neck is of primary clinical importance. Since they are anatomic structures of small size, surface coils

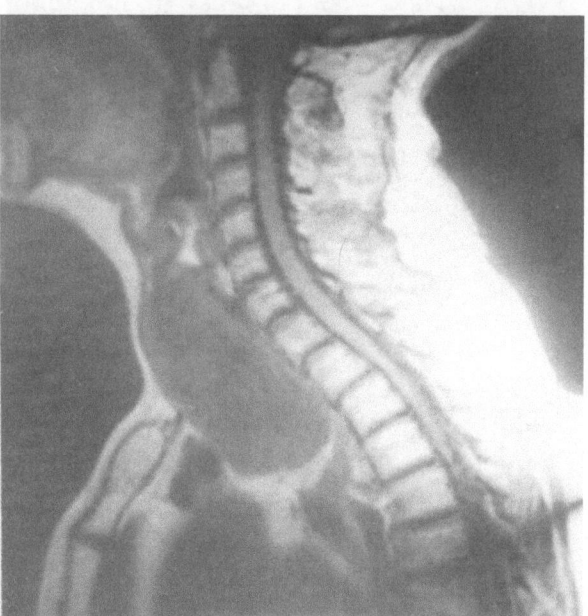

Figure 44. Sagittal T_1-CW image showing a goiter with retrosternal and intrathoracic extension. [Figure 44 appears by courtesy of Dr Gary Stimac, North Shore Imaging Center, Peabody, Mass., U.S.A.].

are required, as well as imaging in the axial, coronal, and occasionally in the sagittal planes, with at least one set of T_2-CW images. Their signal characteristics are intermediate SI on T_1-CW images and high, but also intermediate SI on T_2-CW images, depending on the histological features of the lymph node. The criterion of size (equal or superior to 15 mm in diameter for the submandibular and jugulodigastric regions, equal or superior to 10 mm for cervical lymph nodes of other regions) is one of the most reliable predictors of their pathological nature [40]. Necrosis of lymph nodes, commonly seen in metastatic squamous cell carcinoma, is detected on MR T_2-CW images by high SI, but cannot be differentiated from high SI reactive lymph nodes. However, CT, in such instances, provides more definitive information by showing the low attenuation areas of the necrotic nodes and the extranodal spread [41].

4.4 Gadolinium-DTPA for MR imaging in the head and neck

Paramagnetic substances shorten the relaxation times of tissue in which they reside. This accounts for the high SI observed on T_1-CW images.

Some paramagnetic substances, such as degradation products of hemoglobin, are by-products of pathological tissue changes. Contrast media with paramagnetic properties enhance lesions (or part of a lesion) that have poor contrast *vis-à-vis* the surrounding tissue; thus making them easily detectable on MR images.

The substance used for examination in humans is Gadolinium-diethylene-triamine penta-acetic acid (Gd-DTPA), administered by intravenous administration. Like iodinated contrast media, it produces enhancement of vascular tumors by diffusion, and

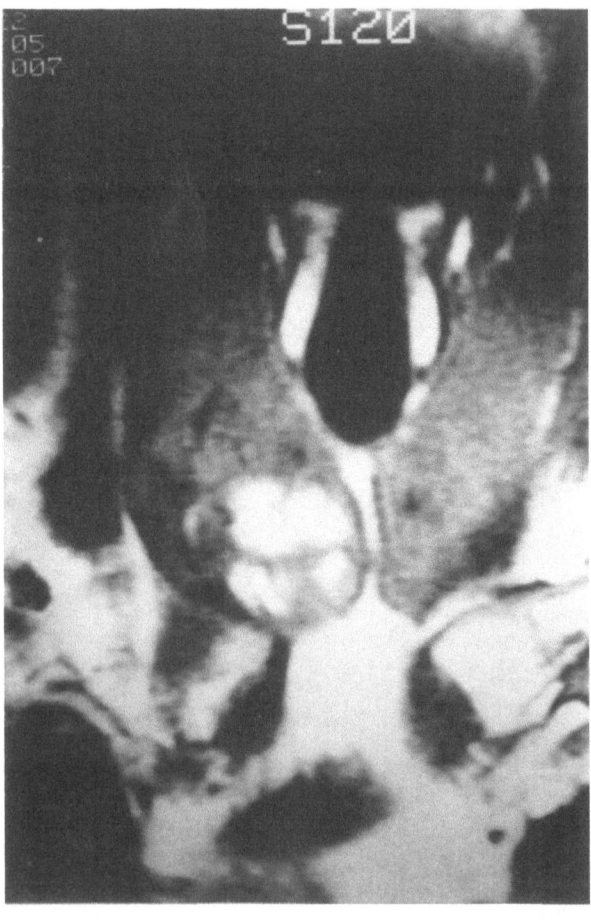

Figure 45. Coronal T_1-CW image of multinodular goiter with areas of cystic change and colloid accumulation reflected by high SI.

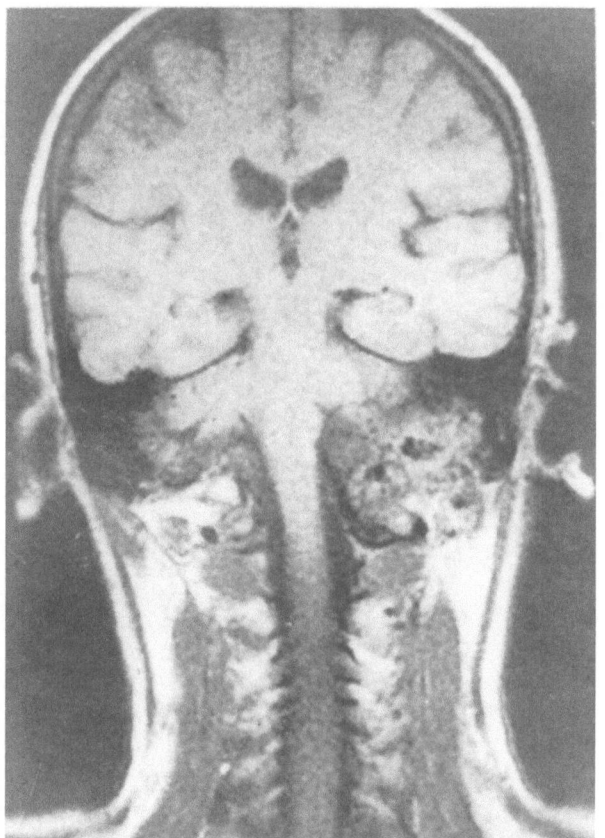
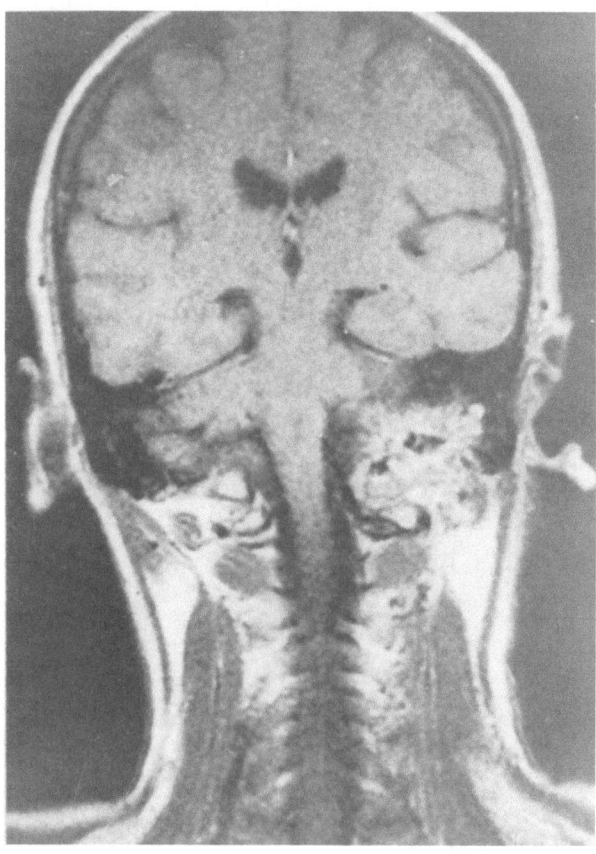

A   B

Figure 46. *Left glomus jugulare tumor.* (**A**) *Coronal T_1-CW image through both posterior aspects of the temporal bone* reveals a large mass with intermediate SI. Note the signal void areas within the tumor reflecting vascular channels. There is erosion of the jugular fossa and adjacent mastoid, superiorly. The tumor extends into the upper neck, and medially, into the subarachnoid space at the junction between the cerebellum and medulla. (**B**) *Following the administration of Gd-DTPA*, there is diffuse enhancement of the lesion which is better delineated. Note again the signal void areas reflecting hypervascularity. [Fig. 46A & B appear by courtesy of Dr Friedhelm Zanella, Radiological Institute of Cologne, Cologne, F.R.G.].

penetrates a disrupted blood–brain barrier. No serious adverse effects (allergic reactions, in particular), have been observed so far.

On a T_1-CW image, SI increases in a lesion harboring Gadolinium-DTPA. Standard SE and fast imaging GRE pulse sequences producing T_1-CW images are obtained before, and 3–4 minutes after bolus injection. The adminstered dose is usually 0.1 micromole per kg [8].

In patients with extracranial lesions of the head and neck, this signal enhancement of a tumor is often helpful in demonstrating paragangliomas [21] (Figure 46) and acoustic neurinomas [17], and is also very useful to better visualize and delineate naso-pharyngeal carcinomas [42], tumors of the nasal cavity and paranasal sinuses and tumors having peri-neural or intracranial extension [43]. Tumors of the tongue and oropharynx (Figures 47 & 48) show moderate enhancement but improved tissue tumor contrast [8, 43].

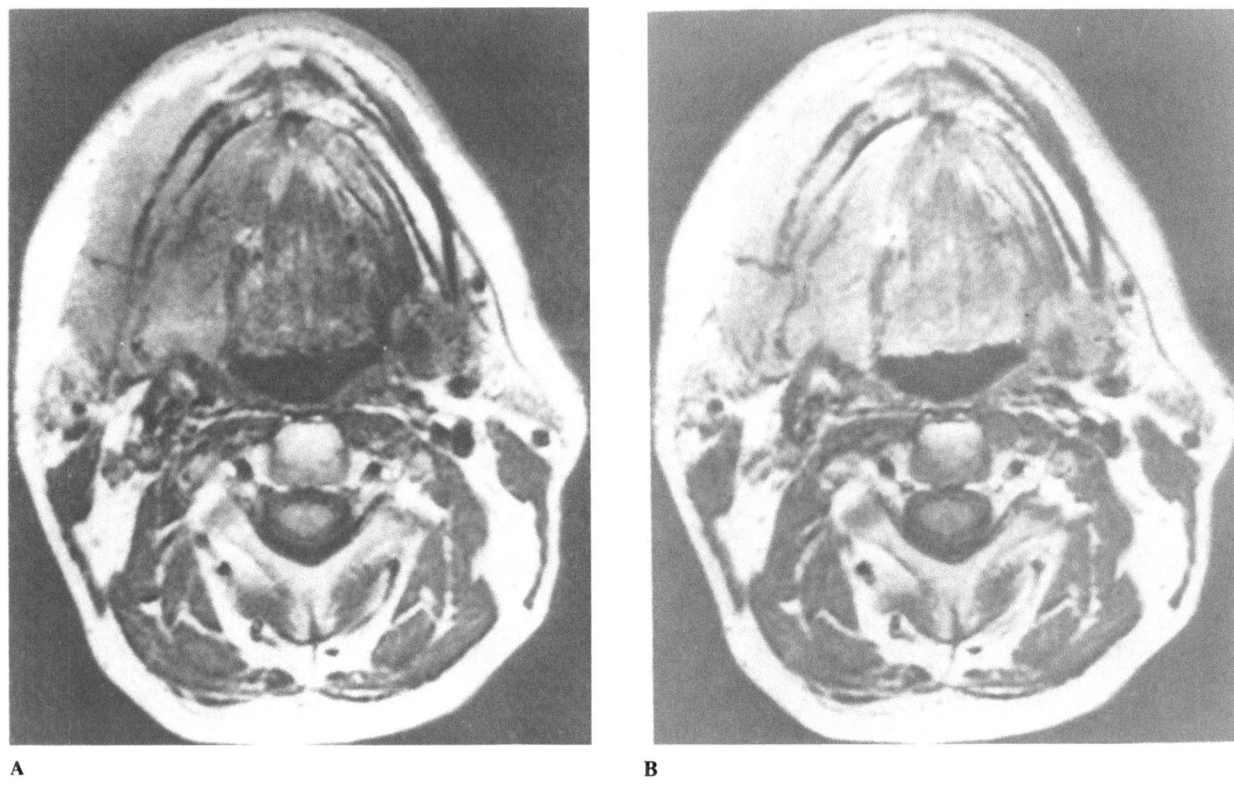

A   B

Figure 47. *Carcinoma of the right oral cavity with mandibular invasion.* (**A**) *Axial T₁-CW image at the level of the oral cavity and adjacent mandible* reveals a mass in the floor of the mouth on the right with extension to the adjacent tongue. There is invasion of the body and ascending ramus of the mandible, which is indicated by obliteration of the normal high SI, fatty bone marrow. There is interruption of the signal void of the inner and outer cortex of the mandible. The tumor extends lateral to the mandible into the adjacent soft tissue structures. Part of the subcutaneous fat is invaded by the tumor, which is best appreciated when compared with the left side. (**B**) *Axial image at the same level post Gadolinium injection* reveals diffuse enhancement of the lesion with consequent better delineation of the tumor boundaries, especially at the posterior margin.

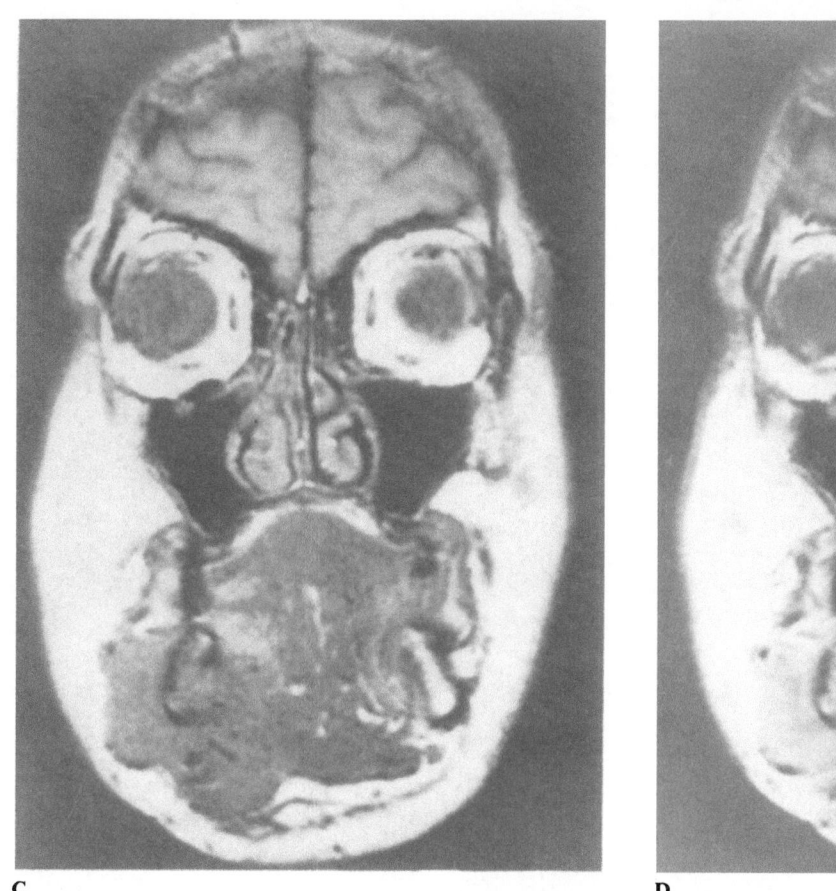

C

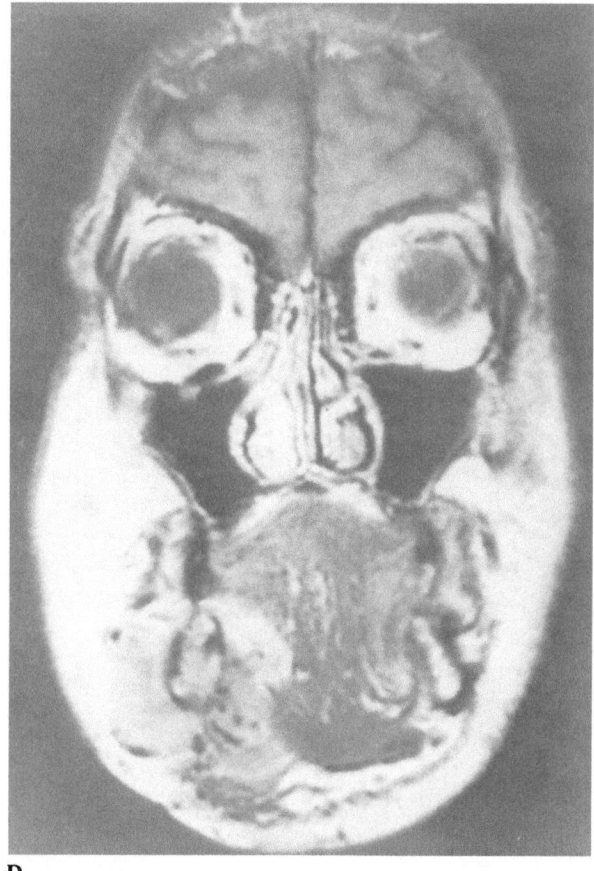

D

Figure 47. **(C)** *Coronal T_1 -CW image at the level of the mid portion of the oral cavity* demonstrates tumor of intermediate SI extending from the oral cavity on the right inferiorly, with invasion of the immediate subcutaneous fatty tissue. There is also extension of tumor into the mandible and soft tissues lateral to the mandible. This mandibular invasion is characterized by obliteration of the fat within the bone marrow and interruption of the signal void cortex. **(D)** *Coronal image at the same level following Gadolinium injection* reveals marked enhancement of the tumor with better definition of the boundaries, especially medially at the interface with the tongue. The tongue is invaded inferiorly near the floor of the mouth.

[Fig. 47A, B, C, D appear by courtesy of Dr Friedhelm Zanella, Radiological Institute of Cologne, Cologne, F.R.G.].

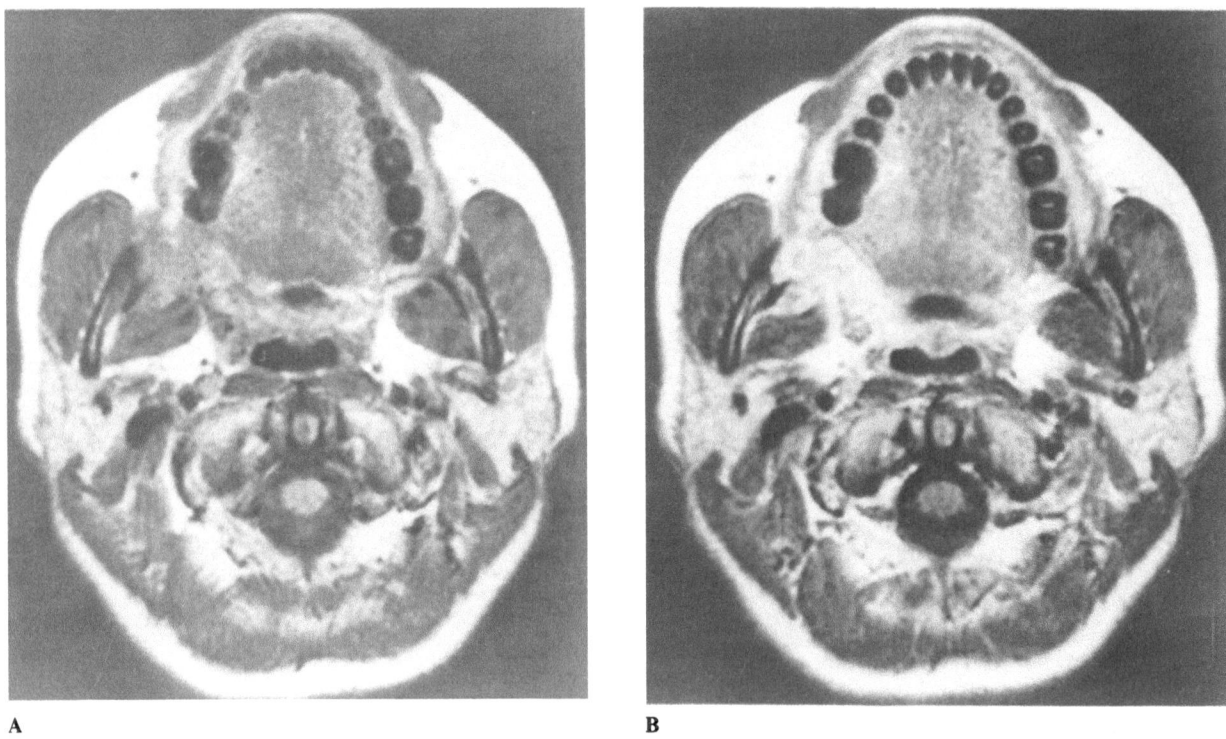

A   B

Figure 48. *Synovial sarcoma in the right anterior masticator space* . (**A**) *Axial T_1-CW image* reveals an intermediate SI mass in the anterior masticator space anterior and medial to the pterygoid muscle and mandible, respectively. The pterygoid muscle is slightly displaced medially and posteriorly. There is a suggestion of invasion of the anterior border of the ascending ramus of the mandible. This invasion is reflected by loss of cortex signal void. The tumor extends to the maxilla and adjacent hard palate, and posteriorly to the third right maxillary molar tooth. (**B**) *Axial image at the same level as (A) following the administration of Gd-DTPA* shows diffuse enhancement of this lesion. Note the better delineation of the anterior medial boundary against the hard palate and of the invasion into the anterior cortex of the ascending ramus of the right mandible.

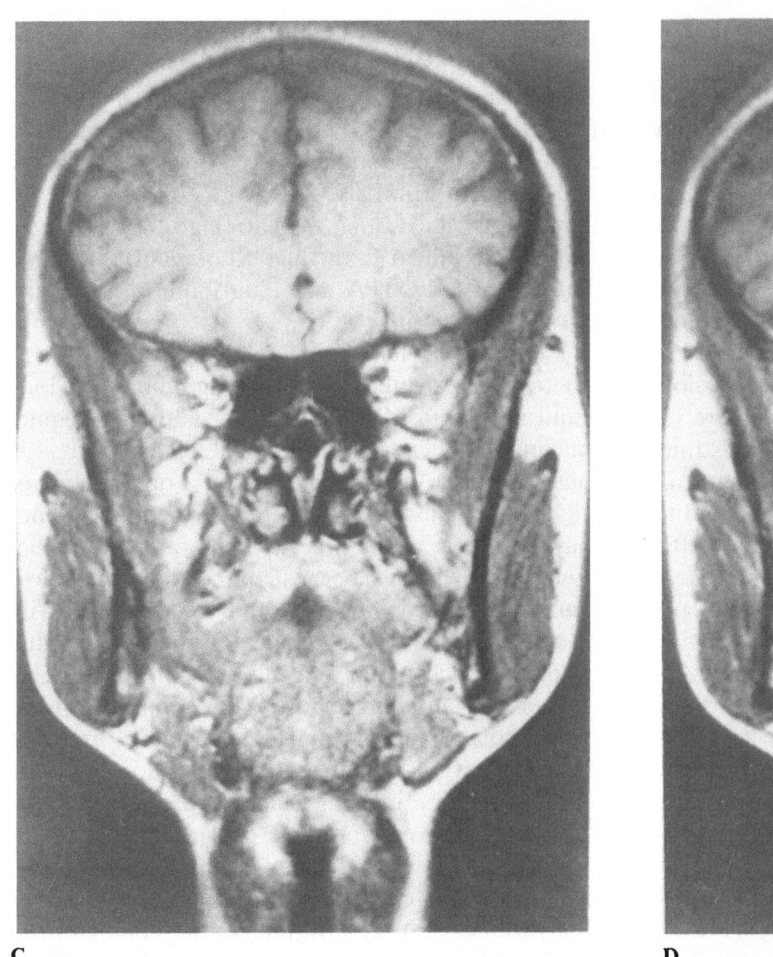

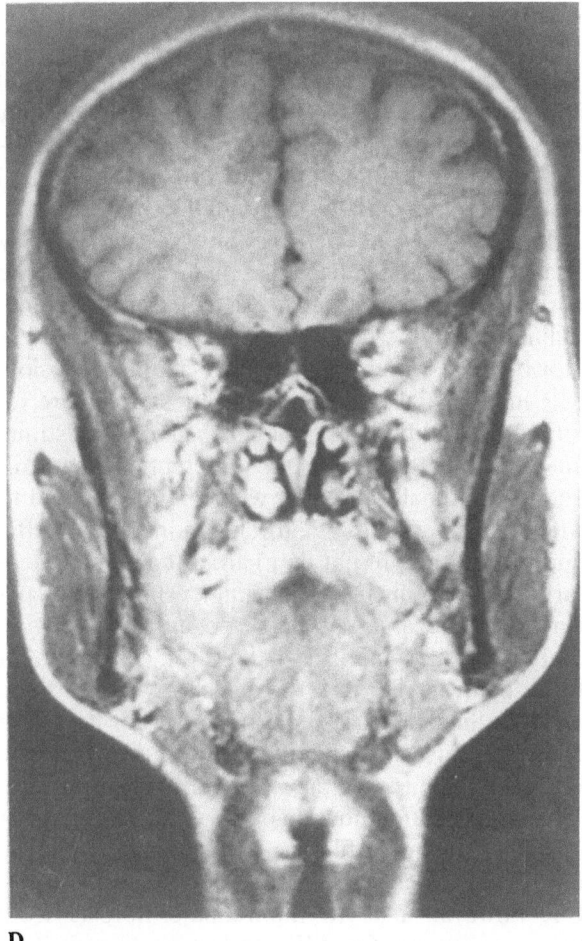

C

D

Figure 48. (**C**) *T$_1$-CW coronal image at the level of the oral cavity* reveals a tumor of intermediate SI in the right masticator space with extension to the hard palate and lateral wall of the oropharynx. The tumor is not well circumscribed on this image. (**D**) *Coronal image at the same level as* (C) *following administration of Gadolinium* shows marked enhancement of the tumor. The invasion of the mandible is clearly reflected by loss of the signal void of the medial cortex with a suggestion of invasion of the medullary part of the ascending ramus of the right mandible.

[Fig. 48A, B, C, D appear by courtesy of Dr Friedhelm Zanella, Radiological Institute of Cologne, Cologne, F.R.G.].

4.5 Unresolved problems

There are still unresolved problems in the clinical application of MRI. Some of them are especially relevant to the head and neck region, such as optimal bone resolution, differentiation of fibrosis and recurrent tumor, and the length of the study.

In many instances, MRI, on T_1- and T_2-CW images, is capable of detecting tumor invasion of the cortical bone (which has no signal) and of the medullary cavity (which has high SI) (Figure 49). However, in order to recognize minimal erosion, MR high spatial resolution imaging systems are required. In addition, lesional calcifications constitute an important finding in the differential diagnosis, and are optimally detected with CT, as opposed to MRI. Considering these aforementioned facts, MRI and CT (at the present time) are often complementary examinations in the imaging evaluation of special anatomic areas of the head and neck region (Table 4). Some authors [44], however, consider MRI to be equivalent to CT for detecting cortical bone erosion. Since MRI is superior to CT for detecting medullary invasion, they conclude that MR is the imaging modality of choice for bone evaluation.

The early differentiation between recurrent tumor and post treatment fibrosis is of significant clinical importance, because of therapeutic implications. CT, however, fails to differentiate fibrosis from tumorous tissue. On MR, end stage fibrosis (dehydrated scar tissue) has different SI (relatively low on T_1- and T_2-CW images) from recurrent tumor (intermediate SI on T_1- and intermediate to high SI on T_2-CW images). However, SI depends on the stage of tissue reaction post treatment. This is reflected histologically by the gradual evolution of the acute and subacute inflammatory phase to a chronic end stage with fibrosis. The acute and subacute inflammatory stage often displays high SI on the T_2-CW image, similar to the high SI of recurrent tumor. The use of Gd-DTPA may contribute to answering this question [43].

Another problem of MRI in the head and neck, where patients cannot lie for a long time, is the long acquisition time. Most head and neck tumors require imaging in at least two orthogonal planes for assessment of tumor extent and location. For some areas, such as the nasopharynx, three orthogonal planes may be required for a precise pretherapeutic evaluation. T_2-CW images, because of the additional information they provide, are often mandatory. With standard SE sequences, imaging of the base of skull or of the neck requires axial and coronal T_1-CW images and another set of T_2-CW images, which, with most imaging devices, together requires between thirty to forty minutes. A thorough MR study with three imaging planes and one set of T_2-CW images is even more time-consuming.

Therefore, faster imaging techniques have been developed. Unfortunately, GRE pulse sequences that produce fast T_2-CW images are characterized by signal loss due to magnetic susceptibility effects at air/bone and air/soft tissue interfaces, which are numerous in the head and neck. Other methods of

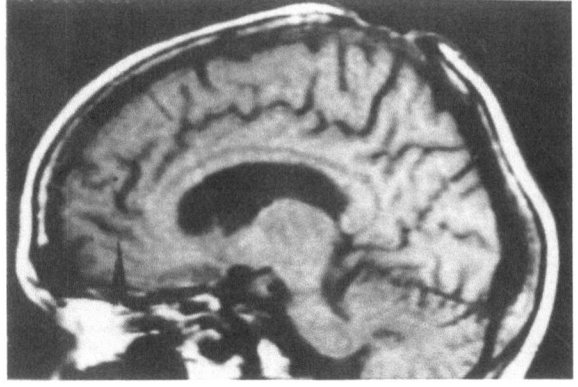

Figure 49. Sagittal T_1-CW image of a squamous cell carcinoma of the scalp invading the fat, subgaleal space, calvarium and leptomeninges. Note loss of signal void of the outer cortex and obliteration of diploic fatty marrow.

Table 4. MRI versus CT in evaluating head and neck tumors.

Orbital regions	MR and CT complementary
Base of skull	MR superior
Temporal bones	MR and CT complementary
Salivary glands/ parapharyngeal space	MR better
Paranasal sinuses	MR usually better, except for bone involvement
Nasopharynx	MR better
Tongue and oropharynx	MR better, especially with Gd-DTPA
Larynx, hypopharynx, and neck	MR and CT complementary

shortening the data collection time, such as hybrid imaging [45] or half-Fourier imaging [46], are currently being introduced into clinical use.

The use of these newer techniques, and a careful tailoring of the MR study to each case, provides the basis for an optimal diagnostic examination.

REFERENCES FOR CHAPTER FOUR: MRI STRATEGY

1. Glazer HS, Niemeyer JH, Balfe DM, et al. (1986): Neck neoplasms: MR imaging, Part I: Initial evaluation. *Radiology* 160: 343–348.
2. Lufkin RB, Hanafee WN (1988): MRI of the head and neck. *Magnetic Resonance Imaging* 6: 69–88.
3. Harm SE, Wilk RM, Wolford, et al. (1985): The temporomandibular joint: Magnetic resonance imaging using surface coils. *Radiology* 157: 133–136.
4. Lufkin RB, Hanafee WN (1985): Application of surface coils to MRI anatomy of the larynx. *Radiology* 145: 483–489.
5. Edelman RE, Stark DD, Saini S, et al. (1986): Oblique planes of section in MR imaging. *Radiology* 159: 807–810.
6. Mikulis DJ, Chisin R, Wismer GL, et al. (1989): Phase contrast imaging of the parotid region. *AJNR* 10: 157–164..
7. Chisin R, Buxton RB, Ragozzino MW, et al. (1989): Preliminary clinical results with low flip angle spin-echo imaging: applications to the head and neck. *AJNR* 10: 719–724.
8. Vogl T, Browning R, Gevers G, et al. (1988): MR imaging of the oropharynx and tongue: comparison of plain and Gd-DTPA studies. *JCAT* 12: 427–433.
9. Som PM, Shapiro MD, Biller HF, et al. (1988): Sinonasal tumors and inflammatory tissues: Differentiation with MR imaging. *Radiology* 167: 803–808.
10. Glazer HS, Niemeyer JH, Balfe DM, et al. (1986): Neck neoplasms: MR imaging, Part II: Post treatment evaluation. *Radiology* 160: 349–354.
11. Ebner F, Kressel HY, Mintz MC, et al. (1988): Tumor recurrence versus fibrosis in the female pelvis: Differentiation with MR imaging at 1.5T. *Radiology* 166: 333–340.
12. Aufferman W, Clark OH, Thurnher S, et al. (1988): Recurrent thyroid carcinoma: characteristics on MR images. *Radiology* 168: 753–757.
13. Bilaniuk LT, Atlas SW, Zimmerman RA (1987): Magnetic resonance imaging of the orbit. *Radiol. Clin. North. Am.* 25: 509–528.
14. Gentry LR, Jacoby CG, Turski PA, et al. (1987): Cerebellopontine angle – petromastoid lesions: Comparative study of diagnosis with MR imaging and CT. *Radiology* 162: 513–520.
15. Koenig H, Lenz M, Sauter R (1986): Temporal bone region: High-resolution MR imaging using surface coils. *Radiology* 159: 191–194.
16. Daniels DL, Millen SJ, Meyer GA, et al. (1987): MR detection of tumor in the internal auditory canal. *AJNR* 148: 1219–1222.
17. Haughton VM, Rim AA, Czervionke LF, et al. (1988): Sensitivity of Gd-DTPA enhanced MR imaging of benign extra-axial tumors. *Radiology* 166: 829–833.
18. Teresi L, Lufkin R, Wortham D, et al. (1987): MR imaging of the intratemporal facial nerve by using surface coils. *AJR* 148: 589–594.
19. Paling MR, Black WC, Levin PA, et al. (1987): Tumor invasion of the anterior skull base: A comparison of MR and CT scanning. *JCAT* 11: 824–830.
20. Daniels DL, Czervionke LF, Bonneville JF, et al. (1988): MR imaging of the cavernous sinus: Value of spin echo and gradient recalled echo images. *AJR* 151: 1009–1014.
21. Vogl T, Bruning R, Schedel H, et al. (1988): MR imaging of paragangliomas of the jugular bulb and carotid body: Fast imaging and Gd-DTPA. Presented at the *74th Annual Meeting of the Radiological Society of North America*, 27 November–2 December 1988, Chicago, Ill., U.S.A.
22. Mandelblatt SM, Braun IF, David PC et al. (1987): Parotid masses: MR imaging. *Radiology* 163: 411–414.
23. Teresi LM, Lufkin RB, Wortham DG, et al. (1987): Parotid masses: MR imaging. *Radiology* 163: 405–409.
24. Casselman JW, Mancuso AA (1987): Major salivary gland masses: Comparison of MR imaging and CT. *Radiology* 165: 183–189.
25. Som PM, Braun IF, Shapiro MD, et al. (1987): Tumors of the parapharyngeal space and upper neck: MR imaging characteristics. *Radiology* 164: 823–829.
26. Som PM, Sacher M, Stollman AL, et al. (1988): Common tumors of the parapharyngeal space: Refined imaging diagnosis. *Radiology* 169: 81–85.
27. Weber AL (1988): Tumors of the paranasal sinuses. *Otolaryngol. Clin. North. Am.* 21: 439–454.
28. Sisson GA, Toriuni DM, Atiyah RA (1989): Paranasal sinus malignancy: A comprehensive update. *Laryngoscope* 99: 143–150.
29. Dillon WP, Mills CM, Kjos B, et al. (1984): Magnetic resonance imaging of the nasopharynx. *Radiology* 152: 731–738.

30. Teresi LM, Lufkin RB, Vinuela F, Dietrich RB, Wilson G, Bentson JR, Hanafee WH (1987): MR imaging of the nasopharynx and floor of the middle cranial fossa, Part II: Malignant tumors. *Radiology* 164: 817–821.

31. Braun IF (1989): MRI of the nasopharynx. *Radiol. Clin. North Am.* 27: 315–330.

32. Brown AP, Urie MM, Chisin R, Suit HD (1989): Proton therapy for carcinoma of the nasopharynx: A study in comparative treatment planning. *Int. J. Radiat. Oncol., Biol., & Phys.* 16: 1607–1614.

33. Lufkin RB, Wortham DG, Dietrich RB, et al. (1986): Tongue and oropharynx: Findings on MR imaging. *Radiology* 161: 69–75.

34. Castelings JA, Gerritsen GJ, Kaiser MC, et al. (1987): Invasion of laryngeal cartilage by cancer: comparison of CT and MR imaging. *Radiology* 166: 199–205.

35. Lufkin RB, Hanafee WN, Wortham D, Hoover L (1986): Larynx and hypopharynx: MR imaging with surface coils. *Radiology* 158: 747–754.

36. Gefter WB, Spritzer CE, Eisenberg B, et al. (1987): Thyroid imaging with high field-strength surface coil MR. *Radiology* 164: 483–490.

37. Noma S, Kanaoka M, Minami S, et al. (1988): Thyroid masses: MR imaging and pathologic correlation. *Radiology* 168: 759–764.

38. Spritzer CE, Gefter WB, Hamilton R, et al. (1987): Abnormal parathyroid glands: high resolution MR imaging. *Radiology* 162: 489–491.

39. Erdman WA, Breslau NA, Weinreb JC, et al. (1989): Non invasive localization of parathyroid adenomas: A Comparison of X-ray computerized tomograpy, ultrasound, scintigraphy and MRI. *Magnetic Resonance* 7: 187–194.

40. Som PM (1987): Lymph nodes of the neck. *Radiology* 165: 593–600.

41. Jacobson HG (1988): Magnetic resonance imaging of the head and neck – present status and future potential. *JAMA* 260: 3313–3326.

42. Vogl T, Dresel S, Schedel H, et al. (1988): MR imaging of the nasopharynx: Fast imaging technique and Gd-DTPA. Presented at the *74th Annual Meeting of the Radiological Society of North America*, 27 November – 2 December 1988, Chicago, Ill., U.S.A.

43. Robinson JD, Grawford SC, Teresi LM, et al. (1989): Extracranial lesions of the head and neck: Preliminary experience with Gd-DTPA-enhanced MR imaging. *Radiology* 172: 165–170.

44. Bloem JL, Taminiau AHM, Eulderink F, et al. (1988): Radiologic staging of primary bone sarcoma: CT, MR imaging, scintigraphy and angiography correlated with pathologic examination. *Radiology* 169: 805–810.

45. Haacke EM, Bearden FH, Clayton JR, et al. (1986): Reduction of MR imaging time by the hybrid fast-scan technique. *Radiology* 158: 521–530.

46. Feinberg DA, Hale JD, Watts JL, et al. (1986): Halving MR imaging time by conjugation: demonstration at 3.5 KG. *Radiology* 161: 527–531.

CHAPTER FIVE

Conclusions

MRI has already proved to be a pivotal imaging modality for head and neck diseases, including tumors. It provides the surgeon with a better anatomic definition of the tumor prior to surgery, and is a guide for the radiotherapist in treatment planning.

MRI, in general and especially in the head and neck, however, must still cope with two major problems; namely, the long scanning time and difficulties in image interpretation.

MRI is not only an anatomical, but also a biological technique of imaging, since the information contained on the image reflects the physiocochemical state of the various tissues that are magnetized. It was even believed, at the beginning of MRI development, that the information on the image could lead to specific tissue characterization and recognition of histologic tumor types. Our work and reports published in the literature confirm the difficulties in determining histology from signal characteristics. More research, such as comparison of MR images with histological findings based on signal intensity calculations and spectroscopic analysis, is needed. The use of a data base bank with collection of large numbers of images, spectroscopic and clinical– pathological data concerning cases with the same histological diagnosis is required for advancing our knowledge of this modality. This method has been introduced in some institutions (KR Thulborn, 1988, personal communication).

In the meantime, MR image interpretation still relies, a great deal, on the morphological criteria (e.g. neck lymph nodes) in the specific clinical setting.

A second disadvantage of MRI is the long acquisition time required for the study. This problem applies especially to the complex anatomy of the head and neck, where multiple plane imaging and high spatial resolution are required. However, MR rapid imaging techniques are making significant progress and should shorten the imaging time in the future.

Other than technical improvements, a better knowledge of magnetic relaxation properties of the pathological tissue, combined with a good understanding of the question asked by the clinician, will aid in the selection of the appropriate pulse sequence, and thereby shorten the examination time.

Index

Index